T0259823

C. Burri   F. W. Ahnefeld

The Caval Catheter

With the Collaboration of
K. H. Altemeyer, B. Gorgass, O. Haferkamp
D. Heitmann, G. Krischak, P. Lintner
A. Ott, H. H. Pässler, E. Plank, D. Spilker, W. Stotz

With 54 Figures

Springer-Verlag
Berlin Heidelberg GmbH   1978

Professor Dr. Caius Burri
Abteilung für Unfallchirurgie des Zentrums
für Operative Medizin der Universität
Steinhövelstraße 9
7900 Ulm (Donau)

Professor Dr. Friedrich Wilhelm Ahnefeld
Department für Anästhesiologie des Zentrums
für Interdisziplinäre Medizinische Einheiten
der Universität
Steinhövelstraße 9
7900 Ulm (Donau)

Translated from the German edition "C. Burri,
F. W. Ahnefeld, Cava Katheter"

ISBN 978-3-540-08566-9   ISBN 978-3-642-66834-0 (eBook)
DOI 10.1007/978-3-642-66834-0

Library of Congress Cataloging in Publication Data. Burri, Caius. The caval catheter.
1. Intravenous catheterization. 2. Vena, cava. I. Ahnefeld, Friedrich Wilhelm. II. Title.
RC683.5.I5B86.617'.414.77-27484.

Typesetting and binding: G. Appl, Wemding. Printing: aprinta, Wemding
2124/3140-543210

Preface

The application of the caval catheter in emergency medicine and intensive care has today become routine. Generally, even in severe shock this route of access to the cardiovascular system is available in order to apply life saving volume substitution. It also permits longterm infusions in modern intensive care, particularly continuous administration of high-osmolarity solutions in parenteral nutrition. In both fields it represents one of the most important diagnostic parameters of circulatory disorders, enabling the registration of central venous pressure. Its undeniable advantages are counterbalanced by the dangers inherent in all invasive methods. Since sufficient experience and precise statistics are now at our disposal, the time has come for a provisional survey. While a few years ago it was considered mandatory to propagate the central venous access in order to advance new therapeutic and diagnostic methods, it is now necessary to reconsider and reformulate indications for its use. In this task it is essential to weigh the expected advantages against the possible complications in each and every case of catheter application. Critical scrutiny must include evaluation of techniques, approaches, and finally catheter materials; this paper presents the results of such a survey. The physician is hereby given the opportunity of being completely informed of evaluating the validity of his standard procedures.

Ulm, April 1977   C. BURRI F. W. AHNEFELD

Table of Contents

List of Co-Authors

Altemeyer, K. H., Department für Anästhesiologie des Zentrums für Interdisziplinäre Medizinische Einheiten der Universität Ulm

Gorgass, B., Rettungszentrum Bundeswehrkrankenhaus Ulm Department für Anästhesiologie der Universität Ulm

Haferkamp, O., Abteilung für Pathologie der Universität Ulm

Heitmann, D., Abteilung für Anästhesie und operative Intensivtherapie des Kreiskrankenhauses Heidenheim

Krischak, G., Abteilung für Unfallchirurgie des Zentrums für Operative Medizin der Universität Ulm

Lintner, P., Abteilung für Unfallchirurgie des Zentrums für Operative Medizin der Universität Ulm

Ott, A., Anästhesie-Abteilung der Städt. Krankenanstalten Nürnberg

Pässler, H. H., Abteilung für Chirurgie des St. Vincenz-Krankenhaus Hanau/a. M.

Plank, E., Abteilung für Unfallchirurgie des Zentrums für Operative Medizin der Universität Ulm

Spilker, D., Department für Anästhesiologie des Zentrums für Interdisziplinäre Medizinische Einheiten der Universität Ulm

Stotz, W., Department für Anästhesiologie des Zentrums für Interdisziplinäre Medizinische Einheiten der Universität Ulm Bundeswehrkrankenhaus Ulm

I. Introduction

When FORSSMANN (169) reported his attempts to sound his own right heart with a rubber catheter in 1929 he met with incomprehension and rejection among his colleagues. Such trials in man seemed too dangerous and unjustifiable. FORSSMANN's superior at the time forbade him to continue his investigations but some decades later his daring was rewarded with a Nobel prize. In the last 20 years catheterization of the heart and central vascular system has developed impressively. Catheterization of the caval veins, the right heart, and pulmonary artery is no longer the preserve of top cardiologic centres but is used widely. The caval catheter today is part of accepted routine in surveillance and treatment, and not only for patients in intensive care units.

This development goes back to the publications of MEYERS (340) and ZIMMERMANN (496) in 1945 who recommended the venous catheter for parenteral feeding of children. For some time after that use was restricted to a few hospitals. In 1958 GRITSCH and BALLINGER (201) reported the successful use of a certain catheter model in 1000 of their own patients and a consumption of over 500,000 PVC catheters in the United States and other countries. In Europe OPDERBECKE (364) published his first experiences with basilic catheters in 150 patients in 1961, drawing attention to the central position of the catheter tip which is now considered necessary. From this time on there was a rapid spread of the use of caval catheters, which in the past decade has assumed enormous proportions.

This recent spread has essentially three reasons:

Firstly the physiologic and pathophysiologic basis was worked out, in the German language zone mainly by ALLGÖWER's group (4, 5, 80, 81, 82, 83, 84, 86, 87) who made possible the interpretation of measured CVP values and thus the therapeutic consequences arising from it.

Secondly, parenteral feeding has in recent years gained increasing importance and widespread use (2, 59, 74, 75, 96, 102, 128, 132, 135, 161, 191, 205, 216, 226, 311, 365, 385, 388, 390, 395, 399). Finally, venesection is no longer necessary for the introduction of a caval catheter with the sets now on the market. The catheters can be introduced by experts without any great demands on technique, personnel, and time (41, 58, 79, 89, 119, 160, 235, 267, 268, 418).

Owing to this development the limits of indications for the introduction of a caval catheter have not only become wider but also increasingly indistinct. We have now reached a point where it is no longer necessary to propagate the caval catheter but to emphasize critical limits of indication in view of the possible of serious and occasionally fatal complications.

When using a caval catheter it is necessary in each individual case to weigh up the desired advantage against possible complications.

On the basis of a study of ours published in 1971 (88) in which nine European clinics and the same number of bacteriologic and pathologic institutes took part, and of knowledge gained since from the literature and our own experience, it will be attempted here — with special consideration of catheter-induced complications — to delineate the indications of the caval catheter, to express a critical opinion on alternatives and possible approaches to the superior caval vein, and to work out statements on catheter material models and the care of caval catheters.

II. Indications for Caval Catheter

A. Caval Catheter in Emergency Situations

In many places the caval catheter is still used only for in-patients. In regions with a well-developed emercency medical service which as an extended branch of the hospital starts its activities at the site of emergency, appropriate treatment is introduced here (Table 1). Under preclinical care conditions special, generally aggravating circumstances must be considered.

Traumatic emergencies and acute life-threatening situations in all fields of medicine, forms of acute circulatory failure, intoxication, anaphylactic or anaphylactoid incidents, as a rule require immediate intravenous administration of potent drugs and suitable infusion solutions. An additional indication for puncture of central veins, unfamiliar to the hospital surgeon, is the inadequacy of arm

Table 1. Indications for caval catheterization in emergencies

1. *Need for rapid intravenous drug administration, infusion and pacemaker implantation*
   in – circulatory arrest
      – anaphylactic reactions
      – anaphylactoid reactions
      – toxic reactions
      – loss of volume

2. *Peripheral vein puncture impossible*
   in – vascular collapse
      – thrombosis
      – obesity
      – inaccessibility

veins in trapped or buried accident victims (AHNEFELD, 3; GORGASS, 194). Since intensive medical treatment with its special facilities, central venous pressure (CVP) measurement, parenteral feeding, etc., is likely to follow, there is only a relative indication for caval catheterization in emergencies when puncture of a suitable peripheral vein is possible. The limitation of this relative indication is due mainly to the fact that puncture of peripheral veins, fixation of self-retaining cannula, and setting in motion of infusion or drug administration take relatively little time, especially when other emergency measures like artificial respiration and/or cardiac massage are required immediately, since even the expert must expect a certain percentage of unsuccessful punctures of central veins. These principles must be observed also in corresponding situations at sites of emergencies outside hospital.

At the site of accident or emergency the possible approaches for the caval catheter are the subclavian or brachiocephalic/anonymous vein, the internal jugular, external jugular, and basilic vein. Since puncture of the femoral vein is hardly performed any more even in routine treatment because of the high rate of later complications and therefore should not be practised under rest conditions either, this theoretic possibility can be ignored with regard to emergency treatment (BURRI, 88).

In emergency situations the time factor is of the greatest importance. The approach to the superior caval vein requiring the least time with the highest possible success rate should therefore be given preference.

The approach to the caval vein system from the cubital veins always takes longer than from the veins of the neck and the subclavian vein, even if the catheter can be moved on without resistance. The fact that the pushing forward of the catheter after successful puncture of the basilic and especially the cephalic vein produces difficulties in a considerable percentage of cases and can then be continued only after injection of infusion solution or abduction and external rotation of the arm, limits the suitability of these puncture sites in emergencies even more.

The pros and cons of the other approaches will now be weighed with regard to certainty of aim and time requirements.

The certainty of aim of a method depends partly on the given anatomic conditions of the approach path with its individual variations but essentially also on the surgeon's technique and experience (Fig. 1). Clearly defined statements on certainty of aim are made in Chapter IV (Approaches to Superior Caval Vein). On the basis of

Criteria for route
of access to caval
vein in emergency

Anatomic conditions
and
experience of
operator

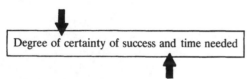

Degree of certainty of success and time needed

Successful puncture
and
pushing forward
and
provisional
fixation

Fig. 1. Criteria for approach to caval vein in emergencies

comparable statements in the literature and our experience the order 1) internal jugular vein, 2) subclavian vein, 3) external jugular vein will be adhered to even at this stage.

As mentioned before, in assessing the different approaches the second decisive criterion for emergency treatment is the time required for successful puncture, pushing forward of the catheter and provisional fixation.

According to experience at the Rescue Centre Ulm, the following times apply to the three remaining approach paths:
Subclavian vein: under 1 min
Internal jugular vein: over 1 min
External jugular vein: considerably more than 1 min
Under the conditions described the three possible approaches may be summarized as follows:

a) Puncture of Subclavian Vein

Despite the at first sight relatively low certainty of aim, as described in our study (88), this path proves the most suitable in acute emergencies in the opinion of the emergency surgeons of the Ulm Rescue Centre.

Reasons:

1. According to statements in the literature, the certainty of aim in several punctures on the same or, if necessary, alternate sides is 93%.
2. The actual time required for successful puncture up to the start of drug administration or infusion is under or about 1 min.

b) Puncture of Internal Jugular Vein

The method of internal jugular vein puncture is tempting because of its high certainty of aim. Allowing for a change of sides a success rate of 95% is achieved. Although the low rate of serious complications in this approach is also impressive, the following disadvantages and difficulties for emergency treatment must be considered.

1. A proviso for successful puncture is careful palpatory identification of the carotid artery. This however is not always practicable with sufficient certainty in people with severe shock, restlessness, and circulatory arrest, in spite of or because of resuscitation measures.
2. Careful palpation of the vascular cord always requires more time than does purely topographic fixation of puncture point and direction with other methods. The time required for this approach is longer than that via the subclavian vein.

c) Puncture of External Jugular Vein

In assessing the approach to the caval system via the external jugular vein two contrary points must be considered:

1. The possibility, in nearly all emergencies, of puncture with suitable positioning of the patient and the short distance to the vicinity of the clavicle
2. The high proportion of cases where the pushing forward of the catheter poses difficulties or where puncture is unsuccessful

The low certainty of aim at this puncture site emerging from our study (88), the high number of cases where difficulties arise in pushing the catheter forward and the numerous faulty positions militate against this approach. The greater amount of time required compared with the other two methods assigns the approach by the external jugular vein to third place in emergency situations.

Complications

Under the special viewpoint of acute emergency treatment a modified spectrum of complications must be considered. Serious late complications otherwise antici-

pated due to faulty position in the venous system, inadequate sterility or the intravasal length of the catheter must be disregarded. It can be expected that after removal of acute vital danger radiologic control of the position of the catheter will be carried out under clinical conditions and, if necessary, another puncture according to the findings.

There are so far no reports specifically listing the complication rate of punctures in the emergency medical service. Owing to the special, aggravating circumstances of preclinical management of emergency patients a higher complication rate must be presumed. Special immediate complications may occur which are partly not yet statistically analyzed because of the small number of known cases. This applies particularly to *pneumothorax* during subclavian vein puncture which hardly ever occurs with the internal jugular vein and never with the external jugular vein. In infraclavicular puncture of the subclavian or brachiocephalic vein therefore an injury to the dome of the pleura under emergency conditions must be anticipated in over 1%. The supraclavicular approach (YOFFA, 494), more frequently chosen during resuscitation and intraoperative incidents because of the quicker approach from the patient's head, is thought even more risky owing to the anatomic conditions. Puncture of an artery may be described as relatively harmless since it is in most cases quickly reversible. In emergency situations, however, it becomes threatening if not recognized at once and if the catheter is pushed forward.

Extravasal positions are possible with all approaches. With observation of the control criteria applicable equally to emergency management (reflux of blood, spontaneous or on aspiration, level variations synchronous with respiration) any extravasal position can remain unrecognized only with preexisting hemothorax and intrathoracic position of the tip of the catheter. In patients under artificial respiration, however, the respiratory level variations are counterrelated, in contrast to those in intravenous catheter position near the heart in patients breathing spontaneously.

We can dispense with a description of signs normally present with intraarterial position of the catheter. In patients with severe respiratory and circulatory insufficiency and peripheral position of the catheter tip in an artery the color and pressure of the blood reflux are unsuitable for the usual differentiation. We know of a case with fatal injuries where in an attempt at internal jugular puncture in deep shock the carotid artery was punctured. There was no cerebral trauma. The catheter tip was intraarterial. After infusion of 6% dextran a wide pupil, not reacting to light, developed on the same side. The patient died of his injuries but autopsy was not possible.

Faulty intravenous position of the catheter tip, occurring with the subclavian vein in 6.6%–9.3%, with the internal jugular vein in 3.5%–7.0% and with the external jugular vein in 12%–17.8%, may be assessed as a relatively harmless complication in emergencies. As a rule another puncture is absolutely necessary only after removal of acute vital danger, when the administration of drugs is possible.

For the prevention of acute catheter embolism the same guidelines apply under emergency conditions as in clinical routine (see Chapter VII, Complications With Caval Catheter).

The danger of air embolism, which should be practically nonexistent under clinical conditions because adequate positioning is possible, must always be considered as greater in an emergency situation. There are two additional points:

1. People wedged in a sitting position, where a negative CVP is anticipated in view of the nature of the accident and symptoms, must occasionally be punctured under more difficult conditions (Fig. 2).

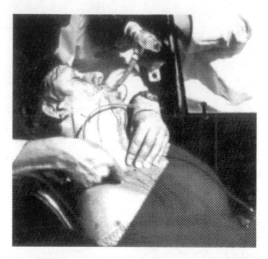

Fig. 2. Puncture of subclavian vein in a driver trapped in a car. While firemen are busy with the technical rescue, doctors and ambulance men are dealing with safeguarding the vital functions

2. In the management of several injured people infusions and infusion systems are sometimes changed by first-aid personnel who underestimate the danger of air embolism on the basis of their experience in hospital and inadequate information.

In this context a case report in the literature is worth mentioning, also the subsequent appropriate animal experiment and calculations according to Hagen-Poiseulle's law. FLANAGAN (168) saw a fatal air embolism in a patient with negative venous pressure of -3 cm H_2O after puncture of the subclavian vein with a puncture needle of 1.8 mm inner diameter. This event was reproducible in the animal experiment. Calculations according to the above-mentioned law showed that a needle of 1.8 mm diameter at a CVP of -5 mm H_2O can pass a fatal amount of air of about 100 ml in 1 s. Although in catheters many times longer the resistance increases in proportion to the length, the danger of air embolism is still obvious.

In the special emergency situations described here the catheter should be clamped before removal of the catheter closure after puncture of the caval system and before changing the infusion system. Under clinical conditions, with the patient lying down and known circulation parameters, this safety measure injurious to the catheter would generally be omitted.

On the basis of the facts stated we can make the following recommendations for the use of the caval catheter in emergency situations.

1. In grave emergencies the puncture of peripheral veins with self-retaining needles should be attempted if it seems likely to be successful in view of the state of filling of the vein, because important complications need not be anticipated.
2. Puncture of central veins for catheterization of the caval vein under emergency conditions should be carried out only by a surgeon who has learned these

procedures under nonemergency hospital conditions.

3. In emergency situations we recommend for the expert in the first place puncture of the subclavian vein, in the second place that of the internal jugular vein (Fig. 3).
4. If a little more time is available, puncture of the internal jugular vein can be tried even in emergencies because of the lower complication rate.
5. In severe states of collapse those with less experience in puncture of central veins should try puncture and, if necessary, short-distance cannulation of the external jugular vein if it is suitably filled.
6. In traumatization of the thoracic region that side should — paradoxically — be chosen for central puncture on which a hemothorax or pneumothorax is suspected. By this procedure additional impairment of the respiratory system by puncture complications is avoided.

B. Caval Catheter in Long-Term Therapy

In long-term treatment the indications for a caval catheter are

1. Parenteral Feeding

2. Measurement of CVP

3. Lasting and Secure Access to Vein

In the pre- and postoperative phase, disturbing factors occur in surgical patients which require early appropriate correction, depending on the patient's original position, the severity of the operation or of the trauma. AHNEFELD (2) distinguishes three therapeutic steps:
1. Substitution of fluid
2. Infusion therapy guaranteeing a minimal diet
3. Parenteral feeding

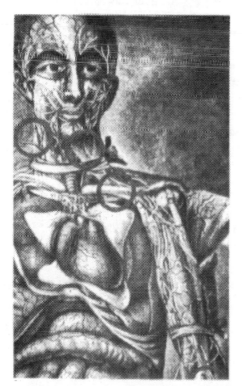

Fig. 3. Puncture routes for caval catheterization in emergencies

Postoperative fluid substitution covers the basic requirements of water and electrolytes. The addition of 5% glucose or sorbit maintains isotony and provides a minimal amount of calories.

Postoperative infusion therapy replaces a minimal diet for 1–3 days. Besides water and electrolytes, 1 liter solution contains 20 g amino acids and 100 g carbohydrates.

If the phase of oral food carence lasts longer than 3–4 days, *parenteral feeding* should be commenced.

What do these facts mean for the technique of the procedures? Fluid substitution can safely take place for a few days via a peripheral vein. Metal or plastic cannulas may be used. For infusion therapy the osmolarity of the solution represents a limiting factor with regard to the mode of administration. The rule is: *solutions up to 1000–1200 mOsm, i.e., a 10% amino acid or a carbohydrate solution up to 15%, may be given peripherally. Any higher osmolarity imperatively demands central administration and therefore a caval catheter.*

Sufficiently well known are the dangers liable to occur with self-retaining cannulas in peripheral veins or on exposing the vein, namely *thrombosis and infection.* The thrombosis may be extensive in isolated cases and lead to embolism, the infection to a septic condition (see Chapter III, Puncture — Exposure of Vein).

Table 2. Indications for parenteral feeding

a) *Primary disorders of enteral food intake*
   e.g., – malabsorption
         – stenosis of gastrointestinal tract
         – extensive resections of intestine
         – tumour cachexia
         – anorexia nervosa

b) *Hypercatabolic metabolic disorders (postaggression syndrome)*
   e.g., – after trauma
         – after major operations
         – in sepsis

Owing to the use of hyperosmolar solutions leading to rapid obliteration of peripheral veins, complete parenteral feeding is possible only via a central vein. TPF has assumed great clinical importance and has been extensively used in recent years. Many questions are still open and controversial. The indications which in our opinion are definite are shown in Table 2.

In the patients of the first group there is a primary disturbance of enteral ingestion. Oral feeding in these cases is only partially possible or not at all. Parenteral feeding is at least partially necessary.

The patients of the second group show severe metabolic disturbance, characterized by decomposition of functional and structural protein. Views on the aim of parenteral feeding in these patients have recently changed. No longer is the supply of calories the main object — amounts of up to 8000 Kcal/day were sometimes considered necessary. The aim is rather to inhibit gluconeogenesis by a simultaneous supply of suitable amino acids and calories in the form of carbohydrates and to promote protein synthesis, thereby ensuring the stock of structural and functional protein (AHNEFELD, 2).

Measurement of CVP. Possible indications for measurement of CVP are:

Assessment of the circulatory situation in cases of loss of volume (trauma, per- and postoperative)

Regulation of volume substitution in preparation for and during major surgery, mainly in patients at risk

Infusion therapy in cardiac insufficiency

Under *artificial respiration*

In *thoracic trauma*

With appropriate measuring technique the CVP represents an important hemodynamic parameter which, interpreted correctly, allows essential diagnostic and therapeutic conclusions. In surgery the information afforded by CVP on the circulating blood volume and the possibility of thereby estimating volume substitution is preeminent. With visible and assessable blood loss, say during operations, the measurement can usually be dispensed with. If volume loss is suspected or not visible and therefore cannot be estimated accurately enough, as, e. g., intraabdominal or retroperitoneal hemorrhages, fracture hematomas, etc., the CVP is an important diagnostic and therapeutic pointer. Assessment of right heart insufficiency, especially in the course of infusion therapy, is facilitated by CVP measurement. During artificial respiration a rising CVP indicates not only the development of right heart insufficiency but also is an early sign of respiratory complications, such as tension pneumothorax. Finally CVP can provide early indications of the development of serious complications in severe thoracic trauma, such as pneumothorax, hemothorax or pericardial tamponade.

Factors raising the CVP are hypervolemia, right heart insufficiency, increased intrathoracic pressure, reduced capacity of the venous system, mechanical inflow obstruction, low position of the head.

On the other hand low CVP is found in hypovolemia, reduced intrathoracic pressure, increased capacity of the venous system, high position of the head, increased cardiac output with cardiac stimulation.

These facts indicate that measurement of the CVP with the catheter tip in the upper caval system (superior caval vein) is a clinically valuable diagnostic aid justifying the use of the caval catheter.

Details about the caval catheter for CVP measurement are given by ATIK (14), BOROW (64), BORST (65), BRISMAN (73), CRAIG (112), DHURANDHAR (125), FRIEDMANN (175), GAUER (184, 185, 186), McGOWAN (196), HILL (234), HOSSLI (246), JAMES (257), JENKINS (258), KEDDIE (269), LANDIS (296), LUTZ (321), MATZ (333), PROUT (382), RYAN (403), SCHLAG (414), SHENKIN (426), STAHL (437), STENGERT (441), SYKES (448),

WATKIN (476), in connection with shock problems by COHN (104), GUYTON (207), HOSSLI (247), LUTZ (322), NAGER (350), PRUITT (383), WEIL (479), WIGGERS (485), and in intensive care by FUCHSIG (179), KUCHER (286), LAVIGNE (301), LAWIN (302), LEVY (309), SCHMIDT (417), SIMON (429), STILL (444), WEBER (477).

The caval catheter allows lasting and secure access to the vein. Limits for the third indication for the 9se of the caval catheter are the most difficult to delineate. To this group belong patients who do not have to be fed parenterally and where there is no absolute indication for CVP measurement but who require infusions for a prolonged period, intravenous medication and often repeated withdrawals of blood daily. A caval catheter in these cases has two advantages that may be important enough in individual cases to justify its use: first, patients whose peripheral veins are soon completely obliterated are spared the torture of repeated punctures or puncture attempts. Secondly patients with secure venous access by means of a caval catheter are much less restricted in their movements than when they have to avoid anxiously any movement with an insecurely situated peripheral cannula.

As already stated, the indications are not applicable without discrimination even in these three main areas but must be applied cautiously in relation to each individual case.

C. Caval Catheter in Children

The first publications on the use of the caval catheter as such, in 1945, came from two pediatricians, MEYERS (340) and ZIMMERMANN (496). They reported even at that time on the successful use of this medical aid in children. But only in the last 20 years has the caval catheter increasingly become routine procedure in pediatric intensive medicine. This is shown by the example of the development

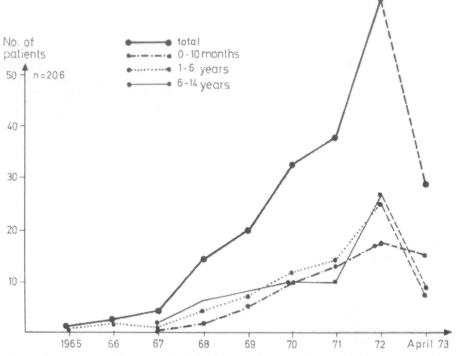

Fig. 4. Age groups and frequency in 206 children with caval catheters (from *Baumann*, 37)

at the Mainz Children's Hospital which may be considered typical of other hospitals too (BAUMANN, 37). But it also emerges from this (Fig. 4) that after 1972 the catheter euphoria was drastically reduced, probably because of the complications encountered. Discriminating selection of indications is therefore required for children, too.

Extensively planned comparative investigations, as in adults, do not exist in the pediatric field. Routine use to an extent that allows comparisons of indications and side-effects is limited to a few centers. On considering the problems of the caval catheter in children it must be pointed out first that one does not deal with a uniform patient material. To mention extremes, a caval catheter may be needed for a premature baby of 1.5 kg or a school child of 50 kg. Sizes from the age of 8 upwards are more or less comparable with those of adults and indications for central venous catheterization are therefore similar or

the same, namely 1) access in emergency patients, 2) CVP measurement, 3) prolonged parenteral feeding with hypertonic solutions and 4), with reservations, lasting secure access to the vein and blood withdrawals for frequently required laboratory examinations. One of the main reasons for introducing the catheter into the superior caval vein is the favorable relation of catheter diameter to vessel diameter. If we assume in adults, e.g., a superior caval vein diameter of about 4 cm and a catheter diameter of less than 2 mm, the distance between the outer wall of the catheter and the inner wall of the vessel with perfect central position is about 19 mm. In the newborn the caval diameter is about 12 mm, that of the catheter about 0.8 mm. The distance between catheter and vessel wall is thus reduced to just over 5 mm, i.e., over three times less. This example shows two things:

The smaller the child, the less favorable

the relation of vessel lumen to catheter lumen, i. e., according to all experience an increased risk of thrombosis.

According to BURRI and GASSER (88), CVP estimation requires an interior catheter diameter of at least 1 mm, so this indication for a central catheter is very seldom acceptable for babies and small children.

Remaining indications in this age group therefore are 1) access in emergency patients and 2) prolonged parenteral administration of hyperosmolar solutions.

Catheter Material

In the introductory publication on caval catheters PVC equipment was used. For children closed caval catheter models of various size are now on the market with tubes mostly of siliconized PVC. Siliconized polyethylene seems even more suitable because it does not harden after softeners are dissolved out. For the selection of the correct catheter size for different ages the general rule is to use the smallest possible catheter for the indication concerned. For the introduction closed puncture is preferable to surgical exposure of the vein because the rate of local infection and therefore possible spread of infection is higher with venesection. The following veins can be considered as possible approaches, without at the moment taking the order of listing as value judgment: basilic vein, femoral vein, umbilical vein in the newborn, external jugular vein, internal jugular vein, subclavian vein.

In view of the special problems connected with caval catheters in children we will first deal with the approaches and complications for this age group.

a) Approach to Caval Vein via Basilic Vein

No great preparations for this are necessary. Very restless children require sedation. If the vein is clearly visible — this is often the case in premature and newborn babies with little-developed adipose panniculus — puncture can be carried out in closed catheter system. Careful disinfection of the puncture site is indispensable. Opinions differ on the use of caps, masks, sterile gowns and gloves for closed system puncture.

After successful puncture the pushing forward of the catheter may cause difficulties as in adults. External rotation and abduction of the arm may make the introduction easier from the bend of the elbow, as may pushing under running infusion or NaCl injection. In babies and small children, surgical vein exposure with increased risk of infection often cannot be avoided. On the basis of findings at the Mainz Children's Hospital, where this approach is chosen almost exclusively, about 90% of 208 catheters via the basilic vein were well placed, i. e., in the superior caval vein. Malpositions difficult to correct were found only in 10% of cases. A primarily ideal position however was achieved only in 26.9% of cases. Therefore radiologic control of the position is required in every case after introduction of the catheter. *If the tip of narrow-lumen catheters cannot be precisely located, filling with contrast media must follow to guarantee correct placement.*

Consequences of basilic vein catheterization, like those of the other methods, may be classified as acute and late complications. Among immediate complications of basilic vein puncture we must mention inadvertent artery puncture, nerve injuries, vessel perforations during pushing forward of the catheter and wrong position of the catheter tip. Artery and nerve injuries are exceptional and played no part in the 208 punctures of the Mainz study. Vessel perforations on pushing the catheter forward occurred twice, i. e., still a rate of 0.8%.

Late complications in the form of thromboses were seen in 4.2% of cases, confirmed either clinically, radiologically, or

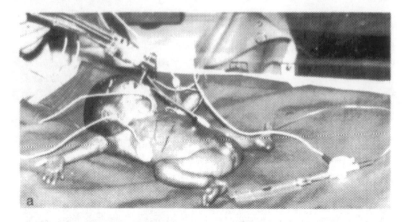

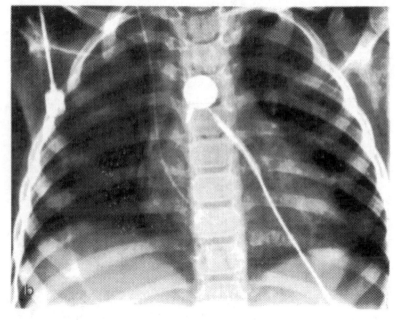

Fig. 5. Caval catheter in a child. (a) Clinical picture. (b) Radiograph showing central position of catheter tip

on autopsy. Compared with statistics of basilic vein catheters in adults the thrombosis rate is only half as high. This result is surprising in as much as theoretically the less favorable relation of vessel and catheter diameter in children should increase the incidence of thrombosis. The cause of this discrepancy may of course be the much smaller number of cases in the Mainz investigations but we are inclined to attribute it to a smaller tendency towards thrombosis at this age.

Infections at the site of entry or phlebitis are rare but exact figures are not available. However, there are records of 13.88% and 10% phlebitis cases in adults, so this complication must be taken into account in children too. Local infections, like thrombophlebitis, depend, i. a., on careful daily attention to the puncture site and above all on the time the catheter is left in position. Sepsis or embolism arising from the catheter were not observed by the Mainz investigators.

b) Approach to Caval Vein via Femoral Vein

Like basilic vein puncture, this technique requires no great preparations. Sedation of restless children is useful. Puncture can mostly be carried out in closed system, so no further measures are necessary beyond careful skin disinfection.

After palpation and localization of the course of the femoral artery the puncture is made medial to it. The catheter can mostly be pushed forward easily but malpositions in the opposite vein or renal vein are possible and radiologic control is therefore indispensable. The catheter tip must lie in the inferior caval vein.

Immediate complications occur almost only in the form of inadvertent puncture of the artery. There are no extensive studies on late complications in children but in adults this approach shows the highest complication and mortality rates, and is therefore rejected. Caval thrombosis with fatal outcome (Fig. 6) has been described in children too (BURRI and GAS-

SER, 88), so we *adopt an attitude of reserve against femoral vein catheterization in children as well.*

c) Approach to Caval Vein via Umbilical Vein in the Newborn

The approach to the inferior caval vein via the umbilical vein in the newborn is conceivable but no longer justifiable because of late complications that are often fatal. Possible irritation of the portal vein may lead to thrombosis of this vessel, followed by portal hypertension with all its consequences. Catheterization of the umbilical vein is now justified only in emergency resuscitation in the delivery room or in exchange transfusion. Infusion of hyperosmolar or strongly alkaline solutions is strictly *contraindicated* because of the danger of late portal thrombosis.

d) Approach to Caval Vein via External Jugular Vein

At first sight this approach appears to be the approach of choice for children. Normally the vein is clearly visible in children of all ages and easy to puncture with the head positioned low and rotated to the opposite side. A roller pillow under the shoulders facilitates the puncture which in small children is best carried out under sedation or general anesthesia. If the puncture itself rarely causes problems, these commence on pushing the catheter forward. DANGEL (115) describes in his summary a failure rate of about 50% in small children. This is quite similar to results in adults.

If pushing forward does not at first succeed, it may do under running infusion or preinjection of saline. This however entails dismantling the closed sterile catheter system. Besides careful skin disinfection, sterile coverage of the side of the neck and the use of sterile gowns and gloves should therefore be practised from the start.

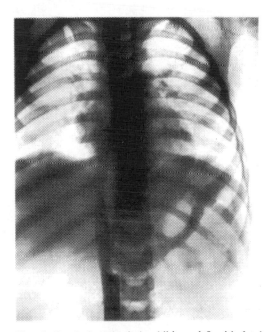

Fig. 6. Caval thrombosis in child aged 9 with fatal result

Because of the relative frequency of malpositions accurate radiologic localization of the catheter tip is absolutely imperative. The incidence of thrombosis in this procedure is 2%–3%. On phlebitis no figures are available; in our experience it is very rare.

e) Approach to Caval Vein via Internal Jugular Vein

In adults this approach to the superior caval vein has rapidly gained in importance since it was first described in 1966. It is also increasingly used in pediatric intensive therapy. Although no exact figures on success and complication rates are available, favorable results easily predominate with this method. An important preparation for puncture is correct positioning of the child and, except in older children, strong sedation or preferably general anesthesia. In view of its straight course the right internal jugular vein is the best approach. In older children puncture can be carried out in closed catheter system and thorough disinfection of the puncture site is sufficient. In small children it is probably better to use the puncture cannula with a syringe attached. Sterile coverage of the puncture area, gloves, and gown are indispensable here. Puncture can be carried out either from the lateral margin of the sternomastoid muscle 2–3 cm above the clavicle in the direction of the upper end of the sternum or by HEITMANN's method (217). After palpation of the common carotid artery the puncture takes place lateral to it and below the external jugular vein. The direction is parallel to the course of the artery at an angle of 30–45° from the horizontal. After successful puncture blood can be aspirated easily but the introduction of the catheter may prove difficult owing to the small size of the vein. Cautious twisting and to-and-fro movement of the needle and introduction with forceps may be advantageous. Retraction of the catheter with the needle in position is strictly forbidden as there is a danger of shearing off and catheter embolism. With all catheters with mandrins, the catheter must be pushed in gently because of the higher risk of perforation in children. Free backflow of venous blood is a precondition for subsequent infusion. The position of the catheter tip must again be determined with the aid of a radiograph and corrected if necessary. The ideal position is in the superior caval vein.

Inadvertent puncture of the neck arteries is the most important of the acute complications. With normal blood pressure an arterial puncture cannot be overlooked and large hematomas can almost always be prevented by compression.

In emergencies puncture of the internal jugular vein should be undertaken only with definite localization of the carotid artery and adequately filled veins. No studies on late complications in children are available to our knowledge, so no definite comparison with other puncture methods is possible. It therefore remains to be seen whether this approach will attain the same importance for children as for adults.

f) Approach to Caval Vein via Subclavian Vein

The approach to the superior caval vein via the subclavian vein is at present probably still the method most commonly used. The puncture takes place in the Trendelenburg position, partly in order to get better filling of the vein but also to avoid air embolism. In children under 8, except in emergencies, strong sedation or general anesthesia is required. The head is rotated toward the side of the puncture whereby deviation of the catheter into the internal jugular vein is intended to be avoided. According to the literature we have seen, the puncture in children is always made below the clavicle. For puncture in small children it is again probably better to use a needle with a syringe attached, and sterile coverage of the puncture area, sterile gloves and gown together with careful skin disinfection are again essential conditions. The puncture site is in the middle of the clavicle, the direction towards the finger tip placed into the jugulum. The cannula is guided directly below the clavicle, according to DANGEL (115) from outside below to inside above. Here, too, the difficulty in small children obviously lies not in the puncture of the vein but in the pushing on of the catheter. Changes of position with rotation of the needle are often necessary but retraction of the catheter with the needle in position is again strictly prohibited. The catheter must be movable without great force because of the greater danger of perforation with mandrin models. Radiologic control is indispensable. The correct position is in the superior caval vein.

A typical acute complication of subclavian vein puncture is inadvertent puncture of the artery. This leads to a hematoma but further arterial bleeding can always be prevented in children by compression (DANGEL, 115). Another serious complication is pneumothorax. In a survey of the Zurich Children's Hospital of 750 subclavian punctures pneumothorax was diagnosed five times, a percentage of 0.66%. Hemothorax was observed three times, i.e., in 0.4% of cases. Catheter embolism or infusion thorax did not occur.

Early complications are inversely proportional to experience in the particular puncture technique, while late complications, provided aseptic technique is used, are inversely proportional to the degree of daily careful attention to the catheter.

Daily change of dressings, careful observation of the puncture site for local signs of infection, clean handling of infusion solutions, and daily clinical examination of children for early signs of general infection are essential provisos for limiting one of the most dangerous late complications, i.e., sepsis. *Since in children, above all in babies and small children, a local infection becomes general much more rapidly than in adults, the catheter must be removed even at the slightest sign of infection.* Normally the catheter may be left in situ for 2–3 weeks.

Infection as the main complication of long-term infusion with nutritive solution is stated by some authors to occur in about 40% but this can obviously be reduced to 20% by strict observance of all precautionary measures.

If the demand for strict limitation of indications for caval catheterization is valid for adults, it is even more so for children.

For a final evaluation of the different approaches at the present time the following statements are permissible:

1. The femoral vein and umbilical vein are not suitable as starting points for a caval catheter.

2. Punctures of the basilic vein and the external jugular vein pose certain problems but should always be used primarily where no experience with other puncture methods is available.

3. The approach to the caval vein via the internal jugular vein and the subclavian vein should be undertaken only with suitable experience, with the exception of some acute emergencies when only the approach via the subclavian vein promises success.

III. Puncture – Exposure of Vein

The possibility of intravenous administration of drugs was demonstrated in animal experiments by WREN and BOYLE (quoted in 418) in the seventeenth century. After the development of the first medically serviceable cannulas by WOOD (quoted in 418) in 1855, drugs were administered parenterally for many decades by injection using syringes. The use of sterile parenteral solutions, disposable cannulas and the development of suitable intravenous transfusion equipment has made infusion therapy possible in wide areas of clinical use since 1920.

Injections

Puncture of veins for the injection of drugs and for withdrawal of blood is usually possible in several superficial veins of the upper extremity, exceptionally of the lower extremity and, in babies, in the region of the cranial veins. How important gentle, careful treatment of the supply of accessible veins is, we have all learned in patients with protracted illness. In the modern disposable cannula with triple-ground tip and silicon coating we have at our disposal a highly developed instrument for single vein puncture (Fig. 7).

Infusions

Based on experience in pediatrics the wing infusion set with short steel cannula, flexible attachments for fixation, and flexible welded-on tube has found acceptance for safe short-term infusions even with difficult veins in adults (Fig. 8). For more

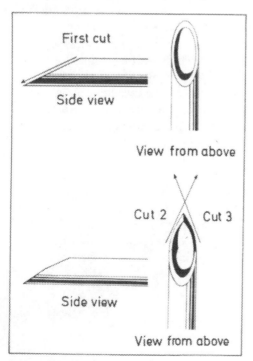

Fig. 7. Diagram of treble-ground tip of puncture cannula

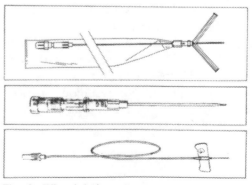

Fig. 8. Wing infusion set, percutaneous puncture catheter with inner cannula, puncture catheter with outer cannula

prolonged infusion treatment flexible self-retaining venous catheters have the advantage of secure intravasal position with greater mobility of the patient.

Self-retaining venous catheters can be introduced as ordinary catheters by venesection and as catheters with inner or outer cannula by direct puncture. Their use as central venous catheters is possible with all the types mentioned. Depending on the approach and duration in situ, however, self-retaining venous catheters in particular are subject to typical and often grave complications.

Choice of Venous Approach

Besides the patient's condition — mainly taking into account the condition of the skin in injuries and burns and collapsed peripheral veins in shock — the kind of treatment required (e. g., high-caloric parenteral feeding, infusion therapy under CVP control for shock, etc.) decides the choice of site and method of venous approach.

The following guidelines may be taken as well founded.

1. Drug injections, blood withdrawals and short-term infusions should be done in superficial veins, of the upper extremity if possible, which are not used as access for a central venous catheter. According to LASSNER (300), the best form of short-term infusion therapy is intermittent intravenous infusion, 12 h per day, with short metal cannula and changes of puncture site of the peripheral vein.

A puncture site should not be used for more than 48 h. In 9.5% of group of cancer patients with baby-wing infusion cannulas in situ for longer periods, Lo-WENBRAUN (319) found contamination of the cannula tip with pathogenic organisms.

2. Long-term infusion therapy and administration of hyperosmolar solutions for parenteral feeding require secure access in a large-lumen vein with adequate blood flow for quick dilution of intima-irritating infusion solutions. In an investigation of 1000 infusion patients MÜLLER (347) showed a clear relation between thrombophlebitic complications and the size of the punctured vein: 11.5% of patients had thromboses in the bend of the elbow, 21.2% in the forearm, 31.6% in the hand and 31.1% in the distal part of the leg. Application of Thrombophob Ointment reduced the incidence in the arm to one-half but had no effect on punctures in hand and foot.

For the treatment and control of critical circulatory conditions a central venous catheter position is required which, besides rapid volume substitution, allows the measurement of the CVP as a crucial circulatory criterion.

Peripheral self-retaining venous catheters are subject to a considerable number of complications if left in situ for more than 2 days, predominantly local thrombophlebitic irritation, bacterial contamination of the catheter tip, local infection, and subsequent septic complications. A summary of nine authors covering 2053 patients (Table 3) shows an incidence of thrombophlebitic conditions of 36% and positive bacterial cultures from the catheter tip in 28.4% with the catheter left in situ for more than 2 days. Bacteremia originating from the catheter was observed in 3.3%.

The summary shows in part considerable differences in the frequency of complications, due to different patient groups, varying periods in situ of the catheter, different catheter material, and differences in aseptic procedure.

Only too often self-retaining peripheral venous catheters or plastic cannulas are introduced under simple alcohol disinfection. This explains the great number of positive bacterial findings. The fact that numerous investigations show a significant increase of complications if the catheter is left in situ for more than 48 h forces the conclusion that all peripherally lying

Table 3. Complications of peripheral intravenous puncture catheters

Author	No. of Cases	Thrombophlebitis	Settling of organisms on catheter tip	Bacteremia/ Sepsis
DRUSKIN (134)	54	30,0%	40,7% (< 48 h 0%)	0,0%
GRITSCH (201)	127	19,4% (siliconized catheters) 42,8% (simple PVC)		
COLLINS (106)	213	39,0%	43,3%	1,9%
BENTLEY (42)	756			2,5% (48 h)
BANKS (28)	118		45,0%	3,4%
KÄUFER (266)	46 (Plastic cannulas > 48 h)	68,0%	53,0%	
FUCHS (178)	364	21,0%	3,6%	
	105 (Plastic cannulas)	21,0%	2,9%	
HORISBERGER (243)	37 ("normal" disinfection)		54,0%	5,4%
	98 (strict asepsis)		12,2%	
CHENEY (99)	135	47,0%	9,7%	

catheters must be removed at the earliest possible moment and after 2 days at the latest.

The peripheral self-retaining venous catheter is therefore inferior to the more complication-free central venous catheter for long-term infusion therapy and parenteral feeding.

Venesection

Venous catheterization by venesection represents a more elaborate procedure compared with puncture, with more tissue traumatization (BURRI, 88; SIEWERT, 427). Ligature of the vein, often practised with venesection, necessarily leads to stasis followed by thrombosis. Deficient washing around the intravasal part of the catheter and inadequate dilution of infused solutions, especially with peripheral venesection catheters, explain the frequency of phlebitic irritation and its consequences.

On comparing catheters via the basilic vein, SCHULTE (421) found complications in 56% of venesection catheterizations requiring removal, against 27% in puncture catheterizations of the same vein. BURRI

(88) in his prospective catheter study found a several times higher frequency of complications with venesection catheters than with puncture catheters – skin irritation in 33.2% against 13.5%, skin infection in 13.5% against 1.4%, thrombophlebitis in 17.5% against 3.4% and thrombosis in 9.8% against 5.5%. Several authors report on bacterial contamination of catheter tips with venesection and puncture catheters and find several times

Table 4. Bacterial complications after venesection and Puncture catheters. Settling of Organisms on Catheter Tip

Author	Venesection	Puncture catheter
FUCHS (178)	25,0%	3,3%
SIEWERT (427)	56,8%	14,0%
BOLASNY (58)	29,0%	6,0%
	5,0% (Strictest aseptic procedure)	3,0%
MORAN (344)	78,0% (Double-blind test placebo group)	
	18,0% (Coverage of catheter and wound with neomycin, bacitracin, polymyxin)	

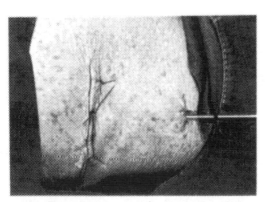

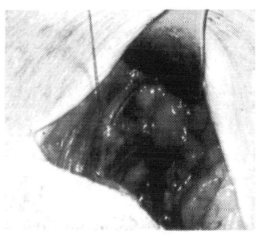

Fig. 9. Bringing out of venous catheter separately beside operation wound in venesection

Fig. 10. Sealing of catheter entry site in the basilic vein by tobacco pouch suture

more frequent positive bacterial findings with venesection (Table 4).

MORAN (344) was able to show that by strictly aseptic procedure and careful catheter management with sterile and antibiotic coverage the incidence of infection can be markedly reduced even with venesection.

An indication for surgical exposure of the vein now exists only in exceptional cases, owing to the various possibilities of approach for central venous puncture. The following guidelines for surgical procedure may be mentioned.

1. That the catheter is led out through a separate skin incision sufficiently distant from the operation wound is a matter of course in general surgery (Fig. 9).

2. The venous blood flow in the exposed catheter-containing vein should be preserved if possible. This can be achieved by
a) Puncture of the exposed vein,
b) Introduction of the catheter into a small secondary branch of the catheter-containing vein,
c) In large veins by securing the site of entry of the catheter merely by tobacco pouch suture (MERKEL, 339; SCHULTE, 421; SIEWERT, 427) (Fig. 10).

Recommended approaches to the central venous system by surgical exposure of the vein are the basilic vein in the upper arm and the cephalic vein in the deltoid-pectoral sulcus. In special cases the approach described by MERKEL and McQUARRIE (339) via a secondary branch of the subclavian vein may be selected. Venesection of the great saphenous vein in the region of the internal malleolus, often still practised for short-term infusion therapy in pediatrics, should be avoided in adults. In babies superior caval vein catheterization can be achieved in most cases by exposure of the external jugular vein.

For the performance of venesection strict surgical asepsis with degreasing and triple disinfection of the skin, sterile covering and sterile clothing of the operating surgeon are a matter of course.

Infusion therapy is an elementary, indispensable part of surgical treatment. Careful preservation of peripheral veins accessible for puncture is therefore of primary importance. Injections and short-term infusions should be done in superficial veins which are out of the question for use as catheter approach. Venous catheterization by puncture is a quicker, more tissue-preserving and less risky method than the more elaborate venesection. As ultima ratio however, surgical venesection is still of importance.

By passing the catheter in venesection through a separate incision, by maintenance of the blood flow in the exposed vein, strict observance of surgical asepsis, and careful treatment of the operation wound and the site of entry of the catheter with sterile coverage, the frequency of complications can be reduced and the venous catheter's function prolonged.

IV. Approaches to Caval Vein

Reliable estimation of the CVP and the possibility of safe administration of hyperosmolar substances demand a central position of the catheter tip in the valveless superior caval vein system. In contrast to other authors (EASTRIDGE, 138, 139; JAIKARAN 256; SAEGESSER 406) and the now very rare advocates of the lower approach from the femoral vein *we consider the superior caval vein immediately before its entry into the right atrium as the ideal catheter position.* If the tip enters the right atrium, complications such as perforations, conduction disturbances, and flat wall injuries may result. Access to the caval vein can be made by puncture or exposure of peripheral veins, namely:

1. The basilic vein or the superficial veins of the arm
2. The external jugular vein
3. The internal jugular vein
4. The subclavian or anonymous vein
5. The femoral vein

A. Basilic Vein

Approach by the arm veins is possible by venesection of the superficial veins in the region of the elbow, the basilic vein on the inner side of the upper arm and the cephalic vein in its entire course up to the shoulder. In our experience, however, the cephalic vein is not, as generally assumed, particularly suitable for exposure. It shows great individual variations in its course, size, and condition. It can be found fairly regularly only in the shoulder region in the deltoid-pectoral sulcus. For introduction of a central catheter through a puncture cannula various forearm veins are possible as well as the cephalic but especially the basilic vein in the bend of the elbow (Fig. 11). Here, too, the cephalic vein very often causes considerable difficulties in pushing forward the catheter owing to its small lumen, numerous valves, or the very curved course in the shoulder region. Of the veins in the region of the arm, therefore, the approach via the brachial vein from the basilic vein can be recommended. Since 1958 the basilic catheter has been used by OPDERBECKE's study group (364–367). In 1961 there followed the first publication in the German literature on experiences with 150 catheterizations (OPDERBECKE, 364). Even the certain basic rules were laid

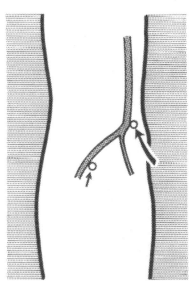

Fig. 11. Access to basilic vein in bend of elbow

down for avoiding complications and their strict observance had the result that the basilic catheter is still preferred by the Nürnberg anesthesia group.

Puncture of the basilic vein takes place after application of a tourniquet round the upper arm, on the inner side of the bend of the elbow, slightly above the joint if possible. After the catheter is introduced through the puncture cannula for a few centimeters the tourniquet is removed and the catheter pushed forward until its tip, after previous estimation of the length (ca. 50 cm), lies in the region of the superior caval vein. In order to avoid perforation of the vessel by the advancing catheter tip, the catheter must be pushed on without using any force. If obstacles occur which may be due to angulation of the vessel or to valves, one must try to overcome them by cautious pushing and simultaneous change of position of the arm. Awkward valves are often overcome by injection of a few cubic centimeters of infusion solution through the catheter or by starting the infusion early and continuing it. If the catheter gets stuck in the region of the axilla, the obstacle can often be removed by maximal abduction and external rotation of the arm and subsequent cautious pushing.

According to general opinion, sterile sets may be used for the approach by the basilic vein. Since puncture in this region is relatively simple, the use of sterile gloves and face mask may be dispensed with. If, however, additional manipulations are indicated, such as injections into the catheter or early start of infusion, sterile coverage of the site of puncture and the wearing of gloves and mask cannot be avoided.

Any caval catheter in situ requires radiologic control of its position. If it is not introduced under direct screening, a standard thoracic film must be taken. Most catheter tubes now in use can thus be located with sufficient certainty without any additional measures. If, however, the catheter tip cannot be definitely seen in the mediastinal shadow, demonstration by contrast media should be resorted to.

More details about the approach by the basilic vein can be found in Brøckner (74), Burri (80–90), Cheney (99), Collins (106), Duffy (136), Fischer (164), Gritsch (201), Hache (209), Henneberg (223, 224), Hentschel (226), Hildebrandt (232), Holt (240), Hughes (248), Ladd (291), McNair (351), Opderbecke (364–367), Ross (399), Schulte (421), Stoeckel (446), and Wiemers (484).

B. External Jugular Vein

Since catheterization of the inferior caval vein was abandoned more and more owing to its frequent complications, the external jugular vein as approach to the superior caval vein has gained in importance, at least temporarily. By the external jugular vein we mean the posterior external jugular vein.

According to Lanz and Wachsmut (298)

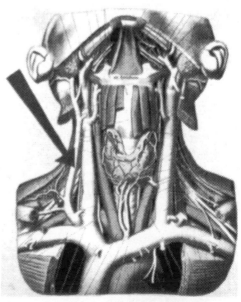

Fig. 12. Topography of external jugular vein

all neck veins drain into the superior caval vein by means of the two brachiocephalic veins (Figs. 12, 13). The three collecting veins are situated in the mediastinum and are subject to the special pressure conditions there prevailing. As in the pleural cavity the pressure in them is lower than the atmospheric pressure. The pressure difference varies with inspiration and expiration between 3 and 5 mm Hg and depends on the position of the body. With the head low, shallow respiration, and small stroke volume it may even predominate so that the neck veins become engorged and swell.

We utilize this possibility for puncture of the external jugular vein. But this inversion of pressure conditions may also occur under pathologic conditions, as, e.g., in tension pneumothorax, mediastinal emphysema, mediastinal tumors, or even merely with violent pressing (Figs. 13, 14).

It is true for all large venous trunks of the neck that they are connected with the

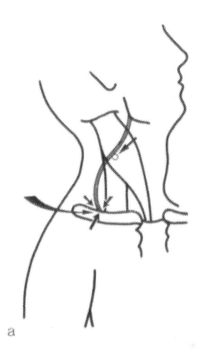

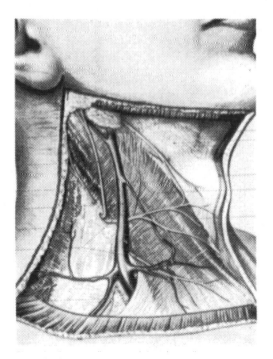

Fig. 13. Course of external jugular vein

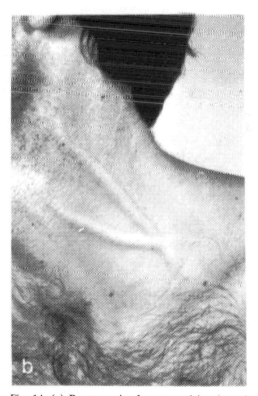

Fig. 14. (a) Puncture site for external jugular vein. (b) By making the patient press (Valsalva) and positioning the head low the external jugular vein becomes clearly visible

mediastinal venous negative pressure which increases towards the mediastinum. The neck veins are therefore pure suction vessels which possess no flow-directing valves for long stretches. In 75% of cases the posterior external jugular vein has two to three pairs of valves in the main trunk, the ventral external jugular vein one pair of valves in 50% of cases. The number of valves in the superficial neck veins increases in a ventral-to-dorsal direction. The posterior external jugular vein drains the temporal and occipital veins of the scalp. It is formed by the junction of the retromandibular and retroauricular vein and runs from the angle of the mandible obliquely over the sternomastoid muscle into the lateral trigone of the neck. Here it penetrates the superficial fascia, reaches the intraaponeurotic space, penetrates the omoclavicular fascia and discharges into the subclavian or internal jugular vein either alone or together with the transverse scapular vein. The posterior external jugular vein is topographically very constant and relatively well developed and easily found even in small children but the thinness of its wall must not be underestimated.

For the puncture in the Trendelenburg position the patient's head is turned to the opposite side when the sternomastoid muscle becomes tense together with the vein. This is made more obvious by compression of the vessel a finger's width above the clavicle and by making the patient press (Valsalva) (Fig. 14). Some authors recommend local anesthesia for puncture of the external jugular vein but in our experience this is usually superfluous. The vein is punctured in the middle of the sternomastoid muscle or slightly distal to it. When blood flows back through the needle into the catheter, the latter may be pushed forward. To be certain of reaching a central position of the catheter, the plastic tube is pushed on for 15–20 cm on the right side and 20–25 cm on the left side.

Here, too, the use of screening is advisable and the central position must always be verified by a standard thoracic film (Fig. 15).

In the approach by the external jugular vein the catheter quite often encounters obstacles in the form of the valve at the confluence or by deviation into another neck vein. If the catheter tip gets stuck in the region of the clavicle or finds its way into a superficial vein, this can frequently be remedied by pulling the arm distally and pressing on the catheter tip from the outside. In any case, the catheter *must not* be retracted through a needle in situ.

We have doubts about the use of plastic cannulas which because of their shortness must lie only in the posterior external jugular vein. This method, often used in babies and small children, can be used in adults during operations only, because in conscious patients there is a danger of perforation by the cannula tip owing to constant turning of the head.

The approach by the external jugular vein is recommended by DUDRICK (135) and others for babies and small children. Further details about technique and possible complications are found in ALLGÖ-

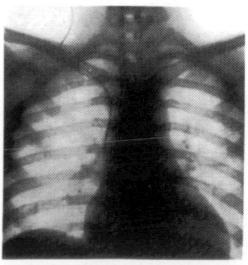

Fig. 15. Correct position of external jugular catheter

WER (4, 5), BORUCHOW (66), BURRI (80–90), DUDRICK (135), DUFFY (136), HENT-SCHEL (226), JONES (265), KEENLEYSIDE (270), McLEAN (303, 304), NORDLUND (358), RAMS (386), SAEGESSER (406), and WIEMERS (484).

C. Approach by Internal Jugular Vein

When we (88) published a comprehensive study on the problems connected with the caval catheter in 1971 there were still plenty of "ifs" and "buts" in the answer to the question of the simplest, most secure, and least risky approach to the superior caval vein, and no patent recipe could be given. The approach by the internal jugular vein, first suggested by HERMOSHURA (229) in 1966, remained largely unknown in Europe and was not even a subject of discussion when the above-mentioned study was written.

The anesthesia group of Erlangen University, especially HEITMANN (216, 217), have earned lasting merit in this procedure. After a visit to the Cleveland Clinic, Ohio, HEITMANN (216, 217) took up this technique and tested it for wider applicability. He postulated three points for puncture of this vessel:

1. As far distant from the pleura as possible
2. As far distant from the arteries as possible (common carotid, subclavian, anonymous)
3. Puncture needle and vein in the same axis as far as possible

Based on these postulates a puncture technique resulted which, in contrast to the divergent suggestions of DAILY (114), ENGLISH (149), and JERNIGAN (259, 260), is characterized by a cranial transmuscular approach (Figs. 16, 17).

With regard to indication, asepsis during introduction and catheter care the previously elaborated and by now generally known rules apply unchanged to the inter-

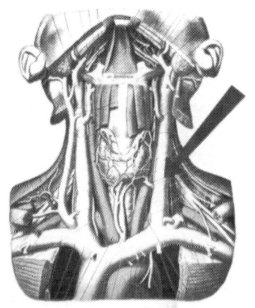

Fig. 16. Topography of internal jugular vein

nal jugular vein approach and must be strictly adhered to.

For safe catheterization by the internal jugular vein we recommend the following procedure.

1. Because of the absolutely straight course (internal jugular vein – anonymous vein – superior caval vein) the right side should always be given preference (Fig. 18).
2. It has proved useful to apply sterile cover on the triangle defined by the fixed points of mastoid, jugulum and the site for infraclavicular subclavian puncture. In this way the approaches by the external jugular vein and the subclavian vein remain available as alternatives if internal jugular vein puncture should prove impossible.
3. Because of better filling of the vein and for absolute prevention of air embolism the puncture should always be performed in the Trendelenburg position, if necessary with the head in the extreme low position, especially in cases of significant volume deficiency and in smaller children.

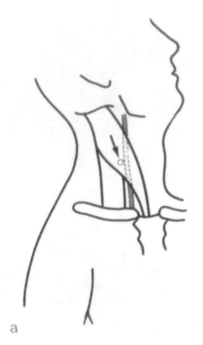

a

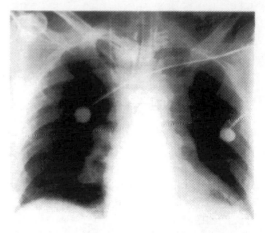

Fig. 18. The straight course of the catheter in the internal jugular vein is easily demonstrated radiologically

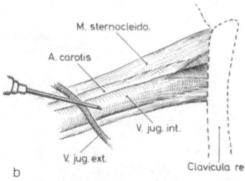

b

Fig. 17. (a) Puncture site for internal jugular vein. (b) Immediate surroundings of internal jugular vein

4. After careful identification by palpation of the carotid artery and the jugular vein under the sternomastoid muscle, easy in relaxed anesthetized patients but also possible with local anesthesia for surgeons practised in the method, the puncture is made transmuscular at the level of the posterior external jugular vein crossing the muscle, at an angle of 30–45° to the skin surface and in the direction of the medial edge of the clavicular muscle insertion. The lumen of the internal jugular vein is reached at a depth of 3.5–4.5 cm in adults, after overcoming a distinct resistance due to the muscle fascia. In most cases the catheter can then be guided without any difficulty into the anonymous vein and on into the superior caval vein.

5. Exploratory puncture with a thin needle preceding puncture with self-retaining catheter is recommended. This is of advantage especially in the very small anatomic conditions in newborns and babies. Inadvertent carotid punctures can thereby be considerably reduced.

6. Introduction of the catheter should, if at all possible, take place under screening control to establish at once the correct position of the catheter tip. Particularly soft catheters of polyethylene tend more towards forming loops which can be avoided or immediately corrected under screening. If screening is impossible, radiologic control by standard thorax film is required.

The following authors have dealt with this approach especially: BAHN (26), BURRI (90, 92), DAILY (114), DEFALQUE (121),

ENGLISH (149), HEITMANN (216, 217), HERMOSHURA (229), JERNIGAN (259, 260).

D. Subclavian/Anonymous Vein

For these approaches the anatomy and topography of the vessels in the region of the superior caval vein are of crucial importance. The subclavian vein collects the venous backflow from the upper extremities and represents the continuation of the axillary vein. On both sides behind the sternoclavicular joint is the angulus venosus. In it the brachial and cranial backflow join to form the brachiocephalic vein, also described as anonymous vein.

Owing to the position of the caval vein in the right side of the thorax, the left brachiocephalic vein is three times as long as the right. The shorter approach to the superior caval vein is therefore on the right.

The right angulus venosus receives the right lymphatic trunk, collecting the lymph from the axillary nodes, clavicular nodes, and thoracic cavity, while the left angulus venosus receives in addition the lymph from the lower extremities via the thoracic duct (Fig. 19).

Two topographic facts especially favorable for catheterization of the superior caval vein should be emphasized (LAND, 294, 295): In the supraclavicular fossa the subclavian vein parts from the closely parallel running artery which turns in a dorsal direction and the subclavian and brachiocephalic (anonymous) veins are connected by connective tissue with the fasciae of the subclavian and ventral scalenus muscle and the medial fascia of the neck in such a way that their lumina are wide open even in marked hypovolemia and the vessels can hardly be missed by the puncture needle.

Four methods have been suggested for catheterization of the superior caval vein from the clavicular region:

1. The infraclavicular approach according to AUBANIAC (15–18)
2. The supraclavicular approach according to YOFFA (494)
3. Puncture of the angulus venosus (235)
4. Direct puncture of the anonymous vein (94, 145)

The puncture site for direct entry into the anonymous vein is between the clavicle and first rib, 1–1.5 cm lateral to the manubrium of the sternum. This technique is generally avoided because of the immediate vicinity of the apex of the lung on the right and the close vicinity of the common carotid artery and the crossing subclavian artery on the left (DEUBZNER, 124).

Puncture of the angulus venosus, e.g., in the subclavian vein shortly before the entry of the internal jugular vein and going in cranial to the clavicle at the anterior edge of the sternomastoid muscle, is also a rarely chosen approach because of the danger of injuring the lymphatic trunk with resulting chylothorax.

The preferred accesses to the superior caval vein are those by the subclavian vein as suggested by AUBANIAC (15–18) and YOFFA (494).

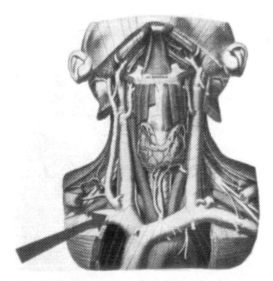

Fig. 19. Topography of subclavian and anonymous vein on the right side

The Supraclavicular Approach According to Yoffa (Fig. 20)

In the method of this Australian author who described it in 1965, a right-handed surgeon should perform the puncture from the left side if at all possible. Correct identification of the sternomastoid angle provides the key to this procedure. Recognition of the edge of the muscle can be difficult in obese patients but is made easier by tensing the muscle while raising the head. If the edge of the muscle cannot be made visible despite this measure, its localization will certainly succeed by palpation. The skin is prepared in the usual way by degreasing and disinfection. The puncture site is at the lateral insertion of the sternomastoid muscle on the clavicle. Here a skin wheal is raised with local anesthetic. The puncture cannula is introduced at an angle of 45° to the sagittal and at 15° to the horizontal plane. The needle perforates the deep cervical fascia and enters the subclavian vein. An intravasal catheter length of 15–20 cm is required to secure a position in the superior caval vein for the tip. It must be borne in mind with this procedure that the tip of the needle is directed from above towards the dome of the pleura and that therefore the pleural space may easily be injured. The pleura is situated only about 5 mm below the subclavian vein and in the direction of the entering needle. Any search for the subclavian vein at a depth of more than 2–3 cm is therefore dangerous.

The Infraclavicular Approach According to Aubaniac (15–18) (Fig. 21)

The method of this author working in North Africa, published as early as 1952, appears especially advisable in comparison with the other methods of subclavian vein puncture because there is a relatively greater distance to the pleura, the direction of puncture — in contrast to YOFFA's (494) method — is more tangential to the pleura, the artery here runs distinctly separate from the vein and the lymphatic trunk is at a safe distance.

For the puncture methods around the clavicle the following points require special attention:

1. Hairy skin areas must be shaved.
2. The skin in the region of the puncture must be degreased and extensively treated with a disinfectant. (Note that the duration of action of the disinfectant determines its effect.)
3. In conscious patients the skin and subcutaneous tissue close to the perios-

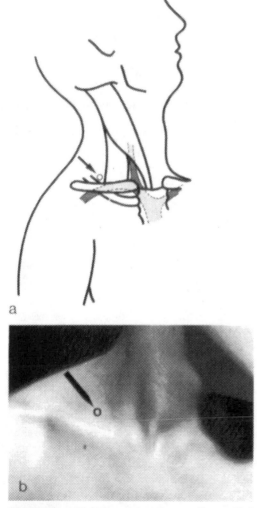

Fig. 20. Supraclavicular approach according to *Yoffa*. (a) Schematic. (b) Clinical

teum are treated with a local anesthetic.

4. The area surrounding the puncture site must be covered with sterile cloth.
5. The surgeon must wear sterile gloves and a mask.

For the puncture the clavicle is the point of departure. The bone is situated directly under the skin and easily palpated. If the puncture is made below the clavicle near its center, relatively few layers have to be penetrated until the vein is reached. Below the platysma fibers and the mostly little-developed panniculus adiposus one encounters first the tough upper leaf of the pectoral fascia which is firmly attached to the greater pectoral muscle, then the lower leaf of the fascia and, after passing loose connective tissue, the vessel. Only if the needle is passed through very closely below the clavicle, the subclavian muscle has to be penetrated in addition to the layers mentioned.

The point of entry of the needle is near or slightly medial to the middle of the clavicle. At the selected point below the clavicle the puncture cannula is introduced in a direction vertical to a line between the acromioclavicular joint and the anterior axillary fold. The vein is reached at a depth of 3–5 cm between the clavicle and the first rib (Fig. 21).

To prevent air embolism many authors recommend, besides puncture in the Trendelenburg position, the use of constant slight aspiration with a syringe. Puncture of the subclavian vein can however be carried out without this aid with ready-for-use equipment where, with the head lying low, blood flows back into the catheter and thus indicates the intravasal position of the tip of the needle. When venous blood appears in the syringe or in the catheter the latter may be pushed forward. Corresponding to anatomic conditions, the intravasal length on the left side is slightly greater, about the same as with the external jugular catheter.

With direct puncture of the subclavian

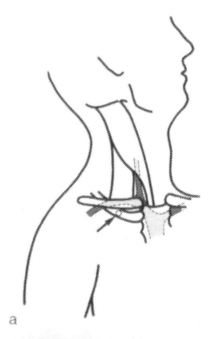

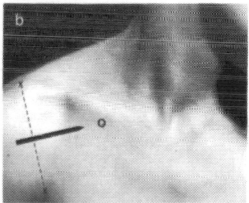

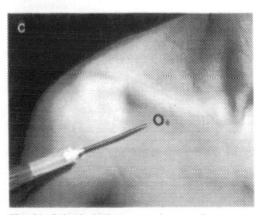

Fig. 21. Infraclavicular approach according to *Aubaniac*. (a) Schematic. (b) Clinical. (c) Puncture site

vein the catheter can mostly be pushed forward easily but with this approach, too, faulty positions are found. Screening or radiographic control are therefore obligatory here too.

On the method of subclavian puncture, difficulties in pushing the catheter forward and complications, there are, besides the original studies of AUBANIAC (15–18) and YOFFA (494), numerous reports in the literature: ASBOUGH (11), BADEN (22, 23), BRADLEY (68), BURRI (88), CHRISTENSEN (101), CLAUSS (102), CORWIN (110), DAVIDSON (118), DEFALQUE (120), EAS-TRIDGE (138), EISTERER (146, 147), ERIK-SEN (150), FASSOLT (151, 152), KEERI-SZANTO (271), KÖSTERS (282), KRÖPELIN (285), KUHN (287), KUX (290), LONGER-BEAM (318), MALINAK (324), PORGES (380), SCHAEFFER (409, 410), SCHOLZ (420), SCHULTE (421), SMITH (430), TO-FIELD (459), VANDEGHEN (467), VOLLES (471), WILSON (487, 488), WRBITZKY (492), and YAROM (493).

TOFIELD (459) suggested a slight modification of AUBANIAC's technique in 1969 which is thought to be considerably safer. According to him the needle must be introduced more steeply near the middle of the clavicle with the patient's head turned away. BORJA (61) takes a more medial approach, i.e., Between the middle third and the medial third of the clavicle and guides the needle in a more horizontal direction. This procedure largely resembles the puncture technique for the brachiocephalic vein. MERKEL (339) described a technique of exposing the subclavian vein in which he introduces the plastic tube through a secondary branch into the vessel.

E. Femoral Vein (Fig. 22)

Among the leg veins the possible approaches for the catheter are the great saphenous vein in the region of the internal malleolus or the groin, and the femoral vein. The great saphenous vein must be exposed in most cases. For adults the method is practically of no importance any more. In babies and small children it is used in exceptional cases.

For femoral vein puncture a pillow is placed under the patient's buttocks, making the groin prominent, and the femoral artery palpated below the inguinal ligament. The puncture is made ca. 1 cm medial to the artery in a slightly oblique and proximal direction. The vein is reached at a depth of 2–4 cm, depending on the patient's physique, and the catheter pushed on into the inferior caval vein.

The use of this method is described by BANSMER (29), BERGER (43), BRÜCKE (77), CHALMERS (96), CHAMBERS (97), DUFFY (136), FIDGOR (160), HOHN (238), INDAR (251), LANG (297), LINDENBERG (311), MONCRIEF (343), POKIESER (379), ROSS (400), TAYLOR (452), and WIEMERS (484).

These are mainly older studies. The method has now been practically abadoned because of its dangers and high rate of complications.

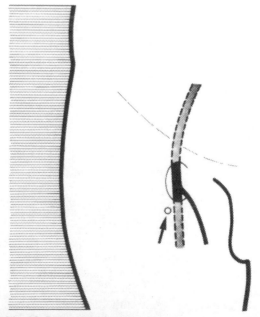

Fig. 22. Puncture of femoral vein

V. General Directions

A. Preparation of Puncture Site

The skin on and around the site of entry must be carefully disinfected with iodine or iodine substitute. Some authors recommend previous degreasing. In HORISBERGER's (242, 243) experience the rate of infection can be significantly lowered, even with the use of ready-for-use, sterile-packed catheter material, by using sterile gloves and mask as well as sterile coverage of the puncture site. If the puncture area is hairy, shaving is of course necessary before degreasing and disinfection.

B. Puncture

This is done in the usual manner. The localization depends on the different approaches described in the preceding chapter. Local anesthesia is advisable mainly for puncture of the subclavian, brachiocephalic, and internal jugular vein in conscious patients. On entering the basilic or cephalic vein one must be sure to remove the tourniquet after successful puncture, otherwise it will be impossible to push the catheter forward.

C. Introduction of Catheter

Using the catheter sets with plastic coating of the catheter tube, which are now numerically most commonly used, the left hand holds the protective cuff at the base of the cannula. The right hand holds the catheter ca. 2 cm away from it and pushes it into the vein. After each push the catheter is fixed against the protective cuff with the left hand, the right hand goes back ca. 2 cm and repeats the movement until the catheter is deep enough in the vein. If difficulties arise at a valve, the protective cuff can be cut at the back end and the infusion connected. With the infusion running or with injection of a few cubic centimeters of saline the catheter can often be pushed on surprisingly well. When the catheter is in the desired intravasal position the needle is pulled back slowly. With split cannulas the needle liable to cause catheter embolism is removed. Next follows the connection between caval catheter and infusion set. Any mandrin present in the catheter lumen must of course be removed first. According to suggestions by various authors and our own experience, careful disinfection of the site of entry or application of an antibiotic spray is advisable.

The puncture site is covered with sterile dressing over the catheter in situ and the compress as well as the catheter carefully fixed with strips of adhesive plaster. To prevent infection travelling along the catheter, the catheter vein and site of entry should be examined daily for signs of irritation. The disinfectant or antibiotic spray should be renewed frequently. At the slightest sign of infection the catheter must be removed. If still required, another catheter must be introduced elsewhere.

VI. Catheter Material — Models

A caval catheter whose tip is correctly positioned in the superior caval vein must be required:

1. To cause as few thromboses as possible (BÄSSLER, 25)
2. Not to be vulnerable to body fluids chemically or enzymatically
3. Not to give off any injurious substances
4. Not only to *be* soft and flexible but to *remain* so

The tubes of the many models on the market (Fig. 23) are made of different synthetic materials. The most commonly used are polyvinylchloride (PVC), polyethylene (PE), teflon (PTFE), polyurethan, silastik (442), etc.

The PVC models easily predominate, the biggest share in the market probably being held by Bard's Model I Cath. PVC, a thermoplastic material, is highly chemically inert. It is produced in very large quantities by polymerization of vinyl chloride. Its structural formula is

$$- CH_3 - \underset{\underset{Cl}{|}}{CH} - CH_2 - \underset{\underset{Cl}{|}}{CH} - \ldots\ldots$$

This substance however exists only as hard PVC and becomes soft PVC only by

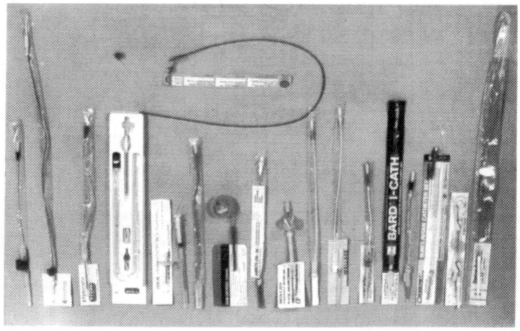

Fig. 23. Selection of catheter models

admixture of quite large amounts of softeners, on the average ca. 37%. Chemically these softeners consist of phthalic ester. They are only mixed with PVC, not chemically combined. In the USA alone up to 500 million tons of phthalic ester are used annually and it is surprising how little we still know about the toxicology and environmental effects of these products. One danger of the softeners arises from the fact that they are relatively easily separated from the synthetic mixture. Since according to present knowledge they are not biologically decomposable (Symposium, Nat. Inst. of Environmental Health Sciences, Pinehurst, N. Carolina, Sept. 1972) there is a danger of accumulation in the food chain, similar to that of DDT (ROLLE, 396; RONK, 397).

Phthalates have since been demonstrated in various American rivers. Early measurements in maritime organisms have shown a rise in these substances to 350–3900 times the normal level in their living space (BÄR, 24).

Acute signs of intoxication after inadvertent ingestion of up to 10 ml phthalic ester were not observed but there are increasing indications of an insidious toxicity of these substances, especially with parenteral use, in the form of disturbances of antibody production, increased vascular permeability, injury to vascular endothelium with induction of thrombosis and, still doubtfully, hepatitis-like liver function disturbance (NEEGARD, 354).

The softeners have a strong toxic effect on cells in the phase of division. For instance, embryonic heart cells die when in contact with serum-containing culture medium previously kept in PVC containers (DE HAAN, 208).

Blood, and especially plasma, can extract phthalic esters from PVC containers and tubes. In preserved blood stored in PVC bags for up to 21 days, up to 7 mg softeners per 100 ml blood have been demonstrated (JAEGER, 255). The synthetic material also loses its flexibility through the loss of these substances and becomes rigid (Fig. 24).

The synthetic substance polyethylene with the simple structural formula

$$CH_3 - \overset{\displaystyle H}{\underset{\displaystyle H}{C}} - \overset{\displaystyle H}{\underset{\displaystyle H}{C}} - \ldots$$

is chemically and physiologically completely inert and needs no additional substances to be made flexible and soft. In contrast to the softening admixture to PVC, it causes no reaction whatever in biologic tissues and retains its physical properties unchanged.

It therefore seemed of interest to us to test the two materials as caval catheters, physically and, with regard to the danger of thrombosis, experimentally and clinically.

A comparison was made between 60-cm-long sterile caval catheters of siliconized PVC and of siliconized polyethylene of commercial origin.

The rigidity of the catheter after being in position intravasally for 0 and 27 days was examined. In 30-mm-long catheter end

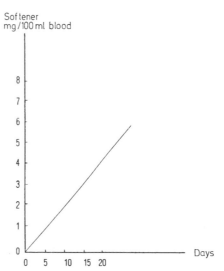

Fig. 24. Softener content of preserved blood after storage in PVC containers (from *Jäger*, 225)

pieces, with constant lever arm and at 37° C, the force necessary to deform the catheter tip was measured in pond. The deforming force required under these standardized conditions increases in direct proportion to duration of the position in situ from 1.6–3.2 pond with PVC and from 2.1–2.4 pond with polyethylene.

In 12 catheter tubes of each kind the sub-aquous clotting-time of recalcified fresh blood was determined in a double-blind test, the test conditions being kept constant. Clotting-time after flowing through the PVC models was on the average 189.8 s, through the polyethylene models 247.0 s. This statistically significant, difference indicates a greater danger of thrombosis with PVC material.

In an alternating series of tests we examined the reaction of the vein to the two materials in 30 patients in each case (KRISCHAK and BURRI, 284). The catheter was introduced into the basilic vein in the bend of the elbow for 5 days, making sure that the tip rested in the vein with a relatively narrow lumen. In order to obtain a genuine result we used exclusively normotonic electrolyte solutions as infusion. A thrombotic reaction was seen in 11 cases with PVC, only once with polyethylene (Table 5).

From this we draw the conclusion that many complications with caval catheters are attributable to the use of unsuitable materials.

In our clinical and physical tests siliconized polyethylene proved superior to siliconized PVC in every respect.

Teflon is one of the fluorcarbon resins and as polytetrafluorethylene has a simple structural formula:

$$\ldots - \overset{\overset{\displaystyle F}{|}}{\underset{\underset{\displaystyle F}{|}}{C}} - \overset{\overset{\displaystyle F}{|}}{\underset{\underset{\displaystyle F}{|}}{C}} - \overset{\overset{\displaystyle F}{|}}{\underset{\underset{\displaystyle F}{|}}{C}} - \ldots$$

The fluorine atom is one of the most strongly reacting known atoms and forms combinations of great stability. This re-

Table 5. Reaction of Vein

	PVC (n = 30)	PE (n = 30)
Thrombosis	10	1
Phlebitis	1	0

sults in an extraordinary chemical constancy within a wide temperature range. *However, the teflon tubes at present on the market show such a high degree of rigidity that their use as caval catheters seems questionable.* According to HOSHALL (245) the thrombosis rate with teflon catheters is higher than with other materials.

Siliconization of the catheter surface is generally accepted because with this covering the thrombogenicity of the caval catheter can be lowered (LEISS, 305).

The structure of the silicones is shown in this formula:

$$CH - \overset{\overset{\displaystyle CH_3}{|}}{\underset{\underset{\displaystyle CH_3}{|}}{Si}} - O - \overset{\overset{\displaystyle CH_3}{|}}{\underset{\underset{\displaystyle CH_3}{|}}{Si}} - O - \ldots$$

The longer the chain, the higher the viscosity. Only the short-chain silicones can have harmful effects. The silicones are distinguished by a low surface tension and belong to the most strongly hydrophobic substances.

The commercial PVC and polyethylene catheters are silicone-coated and *material-induced thrombus formation is significantly delayed* during the first few days (HILDEBRANDT, 232). Later the catheter causes formation of intravasal clots through mechanical injury to the endothelium, due to rigidity or, chemically, through giving off harmful admixtures. This is the great disadvantage of PVC material as compared with polyethylene.

From the mass of catheter models on offer the most popular ones are listed here:
1. The extremely well-known model I-Cath (Bard) is very easy to handle and

has a keenly ground but nonremovable needle so that there is always the danger of cutting the catheter off, with subsequent catheter embolism. The material consists of PVC with a considerable admixture of softeners.

2. Similarly conceived is model E-Z-Cath (Deseret). Again the needle consists of a nonremovable steel cannula and the tube of PVC. Compared with the I-Cath this model has no advantages. Recently a model by the same makers has come on the market where the needle is removable. The catheter tube consists of relatively rigid teflon.

3. Model Medi-Cath (Chesebrough-Ponds Inc.) consists of soft silastik, is aseptic because of the injection chamber but very complicated and almost unmanageable. The needle is removable.

4. Model Vercath (Vermed, France) consists of teflon without mandrin. The cannula has a ventral slit, allowing the catheter to glide directly along the skin at the point of entry. It therefore comes into contact with tissue thrombokinase and possibly even with pathogenic organisms.

5. Model Intrafusor (McGaw, USA) consists of a PVC tube with nonremovable steel cannula. It is very awkward to handle. The catheter tubes (Wallace) consist of extremely rigid teflon material.

6. Model Cavafix (B. Braun, Melsungen) consists of siliconized polyethylene with synthetic mandrin. The cannula has a removable steel needle on the Braunule principle. Needle and catheter parts are separate. Handling is admittedly somewhat awkward but the use of this catheter is recommended because of its suitable material and certain preventability of catheter embolism (Fig. 25).

Taking into consideration all essential facts leading to complications in caval catheterization, we developed our own model in collaboration with synthetics experts, technicians, and industry. The catheter tube consists of siliconized polyethylene, is furnished with a mandrin and is opaque to X-rays (Fig. 26).

The puncture cannula is split on its upper side and notched on the lower side so that it can be split open and thus removed. Owing to a gap on the top of the needle any cutting off of the catheter during retraction is made practically impossible (Fig. 27).

With this model it should be possible to reduce the incidence of serious consequences.

On the basis of experimental and clinical experience we have arrived at these conclusions:

1. Models of PVC with or without silicone cover should no longer be used.

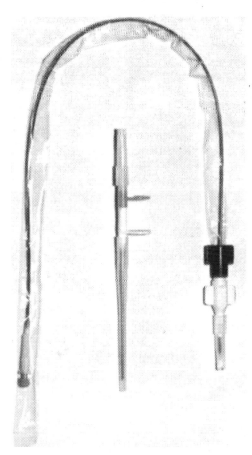

Fig. 25. Cavafix catheter (Braun, Melsungen)

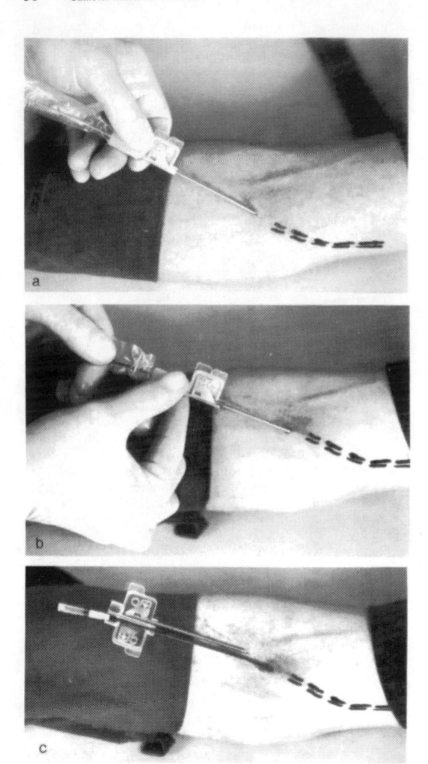

Fig. 26. Technique of caval catheterization, shown by approach via basilic vein with catheter model according to *Burri, Husted-Andersen* (a) Puncture. (b) Introduction of catheter. (c) Removal of needle by opening out. (d) Application of disinfectant or antibiotic spray to catheter entry site. (e) Sterile dressing. (f) Split cannula

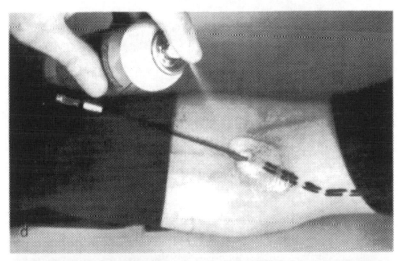

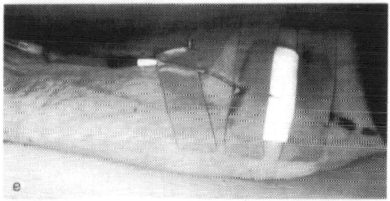

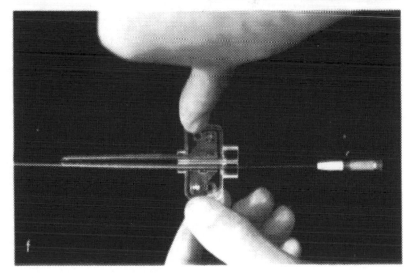

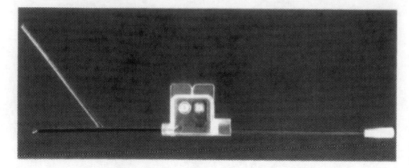

Fig. 27. The model pre-
vents severing the cathe-
ter tube by the dorsal
notch on the needle

2. Those of soft, siliconized polyethylene are recommended as this may significantly reduce the incidence of thrombosis, embolism, and infection because of its tissue tolerance.

3. The use of models with removable needles is advisable.

VII. Complications of Caval Catheterization

The ideal approach to the caval vein is the peripheral vein which is the easiest to puncture and has the lowest rate of complications. We shall try therefore, on the basis of the available literature and results of our own prospective study, to elaborate suggestions for the safest procedure. The numerous statements in the literature concerning these problems offer a possibility from two different sides to classify and assess the complications arising with the caval catheter:

1. Serial compilations with statements on the number of catheterizations from a certain puncture site allow a reasonable quantitative statement on the frequency of various sequelae of caval catheterization. We have therefore compiled 40,058 cases from utilizable studies of 153 authors, including 3241 of our own cases.
2. Description of individual serious or rare complications allows no conclusions on their frequency but shows what consequences are possible and what measures are to be taken if they arise.

A. Complications from Serial Compilations in Relation to the Site of Approach

Femoral Catheter

In Table 6 the results of 16 authors with a total of 658 cases are summarized. In this survey there are no data on the frequency of failures since hardly any of the

Table 6. Complications with femoral catheter (16 authors − 658 cases)

Complications	Incidence in %
Thrombosis	16,55
Embolism	1,8
Phlebitis	4,17
Sepsis	2,81
Death of patient	4,16

studies give information on this point. Wrong position of the catheter is mentioned only by BRÜCKE (77), with 25 out of 100 cases. Inadvertent puncture of the femoral artery has not been described. The femoral catheter however caused thrombosis in 16.55% and embolism in 1.8%. According to the available literature, phlebitis occurred in 4.17% of cases and sepsis in 2.81%. According to SCHULTE (421) who reported on 200 venesections with catheter introduction from the distal great saphenous vein, only 112 catheters were removed without having caused irritation and 88 (44%) had to be prematurely removed because of complications. Six patients died of catheter complications, five of pulmonary embolism and one of E. coli sepsis. These figures agree with the findings in the literature where femoral catheters were responsible for the patient's death directly or indirectly in 4.16% of cases. Important information on the approach by the leg veins comes from BANSMER (29), BERGER (43), BRÜCKE (77), BURRI (88), CHAMBERS (97), DUFFY (136), HOHN (238), INDAR (251),

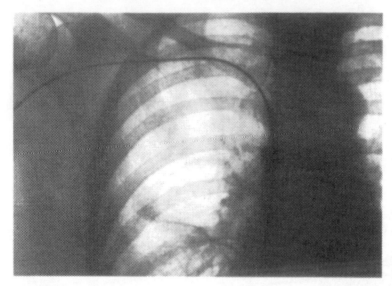

Fig. 28. Correct position of basilic catheter

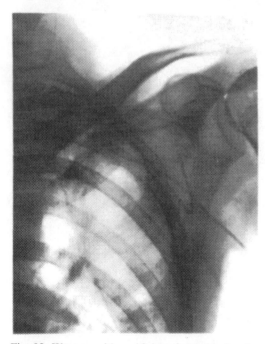

Fig. 29. Wrong position with loop formation in sub-clavian vein in approach by basilic vein

LEMON (306), MONCRIEF (343), ROSS (400), and TAYLOR (450).
This alarmingly high rate of fatal and serious complications obliges us to warn gainst the use of the femoral catheter. The approach to the caval vein from the lower extremity in adults therefore now seems permissible only if all other puncture sites are out of the question, e. g., due to burns or infectious changes of the skin.

Basilic Catheter (Figs. 28, 29)

This approach appears technically simple and some clinics, e. g., the Nürnberg anesthesia group of OPDERBECKE (364–367) who specialized in this approach, report excellent results with it. In the remaining literature however the rate of complications is higher. According to Table 7, accounting for 30 authors with 8058 cases, the puncture did not succeed in about 4% of cases and a wrong position was shown in nearly 10%. Thrombotic and inflammatory complications often appeared after prolonged duration in situ. Clinically manifest thrombosis in 7.64%, embolism in 0.16%, phlebitis in 12.7%, and septic conditions in 0.5% make it doubtful whether this approach should be generally recommended. The incidence of thrombotic and inflammatory complications can however be reduced with this approach too, as shown in more recent studies by HACHE (209), KUROCK (289), and GÜLKE (205). HACHE (209) observed only 3.39%

Table 7. Complications with basilic catheter (30 authors — 8058 cases)

Complications	Incidence in %	
	Literature n = 8058	Own n = 1776
Puncture impossible	4,07	14,1
Wrong position	9,47	16,7
Thrombosis	7,64	9,7
Embolism	0,16	0
Phlebitis	12,70	10,0
Sepsis	0,50	0,06
Death of patient	0,24	0,18

Table 8. Complications with subclavian catheter (77 authors – 20,451 cases)

Complications	Incidence in %	
	Literature n = 20451	Own n = 1098
Puncture impossible	6,18	27,8
Wrong position	5,96	9,3
Thrombosis	0,34	1,4
Embolism	0,04	0
Phlebitis	0,12	0,6
Sepsis	0,49	0
Puncture of artery	1,39	1,0
Pneumothorax	1,08	0,82
Death of patient	0,14	0

inflammatory changes with puncture of the basilic vein but still over 10% with venesection. GÜLKE (205) had an infection rate of 5.1%. KURÒCK (289) had to be satisfied with 15 wound infections and 32 cases of thrombophlebitis in 574 patients and also observed three cases of subclavian thrombosis and one recurrent pulmonary embolism. The basilic catheter was directly or indirectly concerned in the patient's death in 0.24% of cases.

The simplicity of puncture of the basilic vein without puncture-induced complications allows us to state that beginners may continue to use this approach under especially careful surveillance of the catheter. This is the view of the majority of authors who have dealt with the basilic catheter more intensively, such as BRØCKNER (74), BURRI (88), CHENEY (99), COLLINS (106), DUFFY (136), GRITSCH (201), FISCHER (164), HACHE (209), HENNEBERG (224), HENTSCHEL (226), HILDEBRANDT (232, 233), HOLT (240), KLEINSCHMIDT (275), LADD (291), OPDERBECKE (364–367), REICHELT (392), ROSS (399, 400), SHANG (425), VEREL (469), and WEBRE (478).

Subclavian Catheter

The most frequent complications with this approach are shown in Table 8 which comprises the results of 77 authors with 20, 451 cases. Surprisingly low is the failure rate of 6.18% as calculated by us, while wrong positions were seen in less than 6%. In contrast to these statements in the literature the failure rate of nearly 28% in our own series seems alarmingly high. It should be borne in mind however that this was a prospective study which included every skin puncture that did not achieve its object. The retrospective statements in the literature only indicate in how many cases a subclavian puncture was impossible. They do not indicate the number of puncture attempts.

The incidence of clinically manifest thrombosis in the retrospective studies is given as 0.34%, in our prospective study as 1.4%. Embolic complications are extremely rare, as are phlebitic ones with 0.12%. There still occurred septic complications in 0.5%. The four times higher rate of catheter sepsis cases compared with that of demonstrable phlebitis is attributable to the clinically hardly verifiable situation of the subclavian vein.

The gravest complications of subclavian catheterization are acute sequelae due to injuries to neighboring organs during puncture. In the literature we find injuries to the subclavian artery in 1.39% (1.0% in our series) and injuries to the pleura in

1.08% (0.82%). Perforations of the pleura lead to pneumothorax, hydrothorax, or hemothorax, liable to occur alone or in combination (Fig. 30, 31, 32). Deaths due to subclavian puncture can be expected in 0.1% of cases according to the literature. Details about technique and complications are found in AULENBACHER (19), BACH (21), BADEN (22, 23), BAHN (26), BAUER (34, 35), BERGMANN (44), BERNHARD (45, 46), BLEWEFF (51), BORJA (61, 62), BORK (63), DE BOSCOLI (67), BUCHMANN (78), BUCHSMANN (79), BURRI (88), CHASE (98), CHRISTENSEN (101), CLAUSS (102), CORWIN (110), DARVAN (116), DAVIDSON (118), DEFALQUE (119, 120), DIMAKAKOS (129), McDONOUGH (131), EEROLA (142), ERIKSEN (150), FASSOLT (151–154), FEILER (155), FELSCH (156), FONTANELLE (170), FRIEDLÄNDER (174), GALLITANO (181), GARCIA (182), GROFF (202, 203), GULDE (206), HAGEL (210), JOHNSON (261), KAHL (267), KEERI-SZANTO (272), KOCH (281), KÖSTERS (282), KUHN (287), LINDER (312), MAKAROV (325), MEIEL (335), MEISNER (336, 337), NASILOWSKI (352), NIESEL (355), NUGENT (360), OERI (363), PAWLOW (370), PILGERSTORFER (373), PORGES (380), RICHTER (394), SALO (407), SCHAPIRA (411), SCHLARB (415), SCHMIDT (417), SCHÖCHE (419), SMITH (430), SPLITH (436), TITONE (457), TOFIELD (459), YAROM (493), and YOFFA (494).

According to the literature, the approach to the superior caval vein via the subclavian vein by the method of AUBANIAC (15–18) has found the most supporters. Its advantage in representing a safe proce-

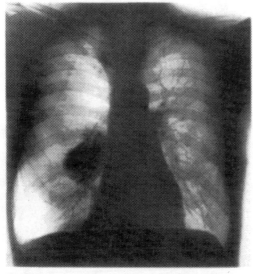

Fig. 30. Pneumothorax after right-sided subclavian puncture

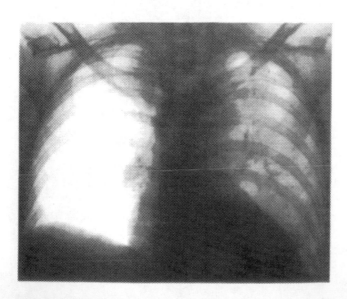

Fig. 31. Infusion hydrothorax with left-sided subclavian puncture

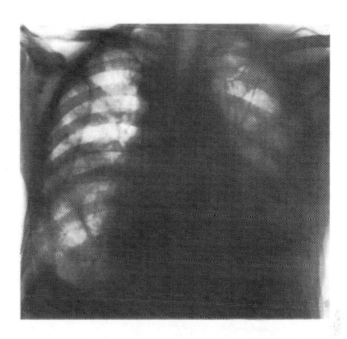

Fig. 32. Hemothorax with left-sided subclavian puncture

dure even in shocked patients is certain. The rate of acute, puncture-induced complications, however, is a warning against recommending this approach to the inexperienced as a routine. Puncture of the subclavian vein should in our opinion be performed only by an expert or in the presence of one. In patients with cardiac or respiratory insufficiency as well as in those with thoracic injuries it is advisable not to attempt it or, in cases of unilateral injury, not to use the unaffected side.

External Jugular Catheter (Fig. 33)

The posterior external jugular vein presents an approach to the superior caval vein involving little risk, as emerges from Table 9 which summarizes the results of 12 authors with 1637 cases. Unfortunately, however, this puncture failed in about 15% and the catheter tip occupied a wrong position in 12% of cases. Careful prospective inquiries produced even higher figures. The thrombosis incidence was found to be 1.8 and 3.4%, with no clinically manifest embolism in any of the pa-

Table 9. Complications with external jugular catheter
(12 authors – 1637 cases)

Complications	Incidence in %	
	Literature n = 1637	Own n = 273
Puncture impossible	14,54	32,5
Wrong position	11,06	17,8
Thrombosis	1,74	3,4
Embolism	0	0
Phlebitis	2,22	5,0
Sepsis	0	0
Death of patient	0	0

tients. The number of inflammatory complications was low and limited to local affections. There was no case of sepsis. So far no death attributable to external jugular catheterization has been described in the literature.

Owing to the obvious puncture difficulties and numerous wrong positions there are only relatively few data on this approach,

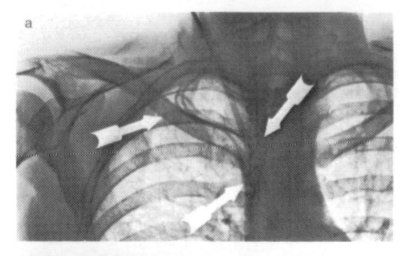

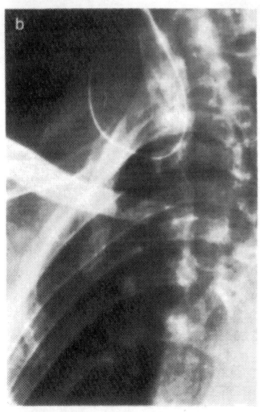

Fig. 33. Wrong positions of external jugular catheter. (a) Loop formation with catheter tip in anonymous vein. (b) Retrograde entry of catheter tip into internal jugular vein

i. a. by BURRI (88), DUDRICK (135), DUFFY (136), GIESY (189), HENTSCHEL (226), ITHOT (253), JONES (264), KEENLEYSIDE (270), KHALIL (274), NORDLUND (358), and RAMS (386).

Internal Jugular Catheter (Fig. 34)

This approach is relatively new and seems not devoid of problems. It is surprising therefore that 17 authors with a total of

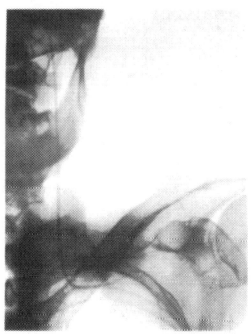

Fig. 34. Wrong position in left subclavian and axillary vein with approach by internal jugular vein

Table 10. Complications with internal jugular catheter
(17 authors – 10,013 cases)

Complications	Incidence in %
Puncture impossible	1,76
Wrong position	0,85
Embolism	0
Phlebitis	0,01
Sepsis	0,01
Puncture of artery	0,51
Pneumothorax	0,05
Hydrothorax	0,02
Death of patient	0

10,013 cases report failures in only 1.8% and wrong positions in less than 1%. Artery punctures with 0.5%, pneumothorax with 0.05%, and hydrothorax with 0.02% can be practically disregarded. In no case did the death of a patient have to be attributed to this approach (Table 10).

According to a recent personal communication by HEITMANN, arterial bleeding through injury to the subclavian artery occurred twice, hemothorax once, and epipleural hematoma once in 3612 punctures. After perforation of the pleural space by the catheter in an 18-month-old boy an infusion hydrothorax developed which was removed by drainage and in one exceptional case, an arteriovenous fistula between the common carotid artery and the internal jugular vein was surgically treated without further complications. Despite long periods in situ there were no cases of clinically manifest thrombosis, nor were any demonstrated by autopsy. In this author's opinion there is probably no doubt that there is a definite connection between the occurrence of thrombosis in the catheter-containing vessel and its lumen and course. The free and straight run of the catheter when the right internal jugular vein is used should hardly provoke any intima lesions, the precursors of thrombus formation.

On the basis of the reports in the literature by ARNOLD (10), BLITT (52), BRINKMANN (71), BRISCOE (72), BURRI (91), McCONNAL (108), DAILY (114), DEFALQUE (122), ENGLISH (149), HEITMANN (215–217), HERMOSHURA (229), JERNIGAN (259, 260), LOERS (314, 315), PAULET-PAINBOEUF (378), and WISHEART (490) and our own experience we have come to the conclusion that the approach via the internal jugular vein under clinical conditions is the one of the future.

B. Complications of Caval Catheterization Outside Serial Compilations

Thrombosis

With the approaches now in use, clinically manifest thrombosis has become a rarity. In stark contrast to the clinical observations however are the findings of REICHELT (392) who on autopsy of 26 patients with basilic catheter found thrombotic changes in the afferent veins in 24. Phlebographic examinations by DIETZ (127) give a similar picture for the same approach. TESKE (453) examined the phlebographic appearances with subclavian catheterization. He carried out 60 phlebographies in 58 patients and found filling defects in the vessel lumen in one-third of the cases. During autopsies of patients of a neurologic department, SABUNCU (405) found mural thrombi be-

tween catheter and vessel 7 times and up to lentil-sized parietal thrombi due to intima lesions produced by the catheter 11 times, also pulmonary embolism in three cases. In ten babies with caval catheters RICOUR (395) found two with severe venous thrombosis and one with caval thrombosis which was fatal. WIRBATZ (489) had to deal with thrombophlebitis in 83% of his cases with intermittent use of the caval catheter. SCHUMANN (422) analyzed 20

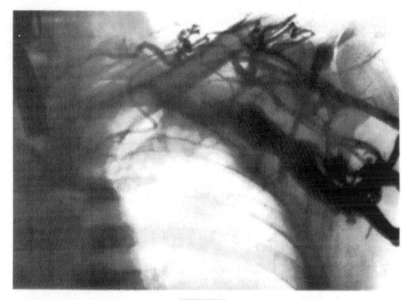

Fig. 35.
Total thrombotic occlusion of subclavian vein with subclavian catheter

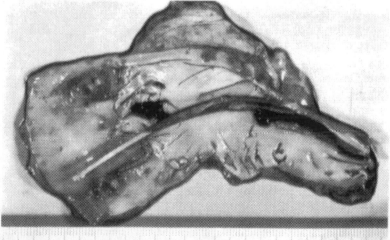

Fig. 36. Ensheathing thrombus of caval catheter in superior caval vein (specimen)

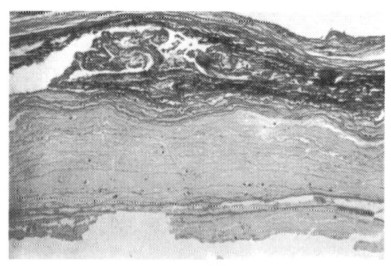

Fig. 37. Histology of same
ensheathing thrombus

autopsy cases with thrombosis and found one thrombus in 6 cases, two in 5, three in 5, five in 1 and as many as seven in 3 cases, four of which were infected. This seems to establish as fact that thrombotic changes occur frequently with caval catheters. With the catheter lying in a narrow vessel the development of thrombotic changes must be expected in over two-thirds of cases, with the subclavian catheter in about one-third. In the overwhelming majority however the thrombosis does not become clinically manifest. Figure 35 shows a case of total subclavian thrombosis after an approach by this vessel, Figure 6 an inferior caval thrombosis in a child after use of the leg veins as approach, Figure 36 an ensheathing thrombus in the superior caval vein found at autopsy, and Figure 37 the histology of this case. Further data on thrombosis and embolism with the caval catheter are given by FFARACS (159), FIROR (163), GRAUDIS (198, 199), HAVILL (214), SCHLOSSMANN (416) and VIC-DUPONT (470). (Abb. 38, 39). The addition of heparin to infusions is said to have no effect on the frequency of thrombosis according to MONCRIEF (343) but other authors saw favorable effects of this drug. In our own prospective study the local tendency to thrombosis was not reduced by therapeutic anticoagulation (88). A significant effect on the frequency of this complication seems to be due to the catheter material itself. According to our experimental and clinical results siliconized PVC causes thrombosis more frequently than siliconized polythylene (92). The latter is therefore definitely preferred.

In our study (BURRI and GASSER, 88) we tried to isolate factors influencing thrombosis formation with caval catheters (Table 11). In patients whose general condition was described as good, thrombosis occurred in 4.3% of cases, with impaired general condition in 8.4%. The frequency of thrombosis was also higher with venesection as compared with percutaneous procedure and there was a definite increase in frequency in the presence of local changes insofar as preexisting thrombosis and phlebitits caused a rise in manifest thrombosis from 6.1% to 20% and 23%. Other predisposing factors of thrombosis formation are previous catheterization, flow disturbances in catheters in situ, and skin changes. There also appear to be significant connections

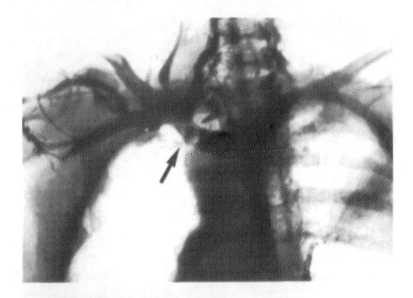

Fig. 38. Subtotal subclavian occlusion

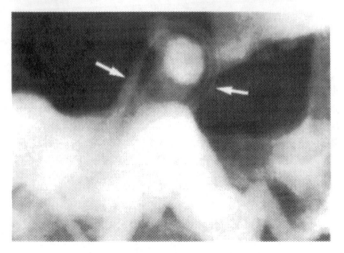

Fig. 39. Thrombus in a catheter loop

between the incidence of thrombotic changes and the point of entry and the duration of the caval catheter in situ.

Clinically manifest pulmonary embolism due to catheter-induced thrombosis did not occur in our study.

If these facts are taken into consideration, if procedures and techniques liable to lead to thrombosis are avoided, if suitable catheter material such as siliconized polyethylene is used, and if the right internal jugular vein is used when there is a choice, thrombosis appears to be largely preventable.

Infections With Caval Catheter

In recent surveys WALTERS (475) reports inflammatory venous changes in 16%, STEIN (439) reports purulent thrombophlebitis in 8.1%, and RICOUR (395) massive suppuration in 1 out of 10 cases. Numerous individual observations of sepsis with fatal consequences due to

Table 11. Factors affecting thrombus formation with caval catheter

Factors	% Thromboses
G. C.: Good	4,3
impaired	8,4
Mode of introduction:	
Percutaneous	5,5
Venesection	9,8
Pre-existing local changes:	
None	6,3
Thrombosis	20,0
Phlebitis	23,1
Previous catheterization:	
Central	6,0
Peripheral	24,2
Site of entry:	
External jugular vein	3,4
Subclavian vein	1,4
Basilic vein	9,7
Others	14,6
Duration in situ:	
24 h	1,4
8–14 days	9,4
36–56 days	11,1
Catheter:	
Patent	5,4
Obstructed	19,1
Skin condition:	
No irritation	2,6
Irritation	19,1
Infection	47,6

Table 12. Serious complications with caval catheter

Complications	n	Deaths
Vessel perforation	41	9
Heart perforation	41	34
Air embolism	24	4

catheterization had been made before 1970, including the studies of MONCRIEF (343) with 4 cases out of 91 femoral catheterizations and of KRÖPELIN (285) with 5 out of 10 subclavian catheterizations. With the latter author this was the outcome of using a selected material of old patients, all under broad-spectrum antibiotic treatment. Of the 5 patients, 3 had a blastomycetic sepsis. STEIN (439) lost 7 out of 295 patients with burns with catheter-induced sepsis, RICOUR (395) 2 out of 10 babies. GENSTER (187) intro-

duced 600 catheters via the basilic and great saphenous vein by venesection. In 33.3% of these cases blood cultures were positive and in 16.4% the clinical picture of septicemia developed. Among causative organisms hemolytic Staphylococcus aureus was predominant, others were Pseudomonas, Coli, Klebsiella, Streptococci, Staphylococcus albus, and Candida albicans. GORCE (192, 193) observed 12 cases of septic conditions with enterobacteria in children. Other observations of local infections are found in BOECKMANN (57), COLLIN (105), FREEMANN (172, 173), KONOLD (283), NORDEN (357), and ORESTANO (368). Several authors tried to pay greater attention to the problem of bacterial contamination with caval catheters. Even with simple cardiac catheterization, with or without angiocardioraphy, bacteremia is said to occur in 4%–18% of cases. Bacteremia has been found in 40% of cases after vigorous tooth-brushing. WILMORE and DUDRICK (486) examined 13 catheters in children, in situ for 6–52 days, 4 of them more than a month, and were unable to demonstrate bacterial contamination in any of the cases. They paid particular attention to catheter care, disinfected the point of entry with iodine, applied antibiotic ointment to the point of entry after introduction of the catheter, and carried out a daily change of dressings. DRUSKIN and SIEGEL (134) examined the bacterial component of caval catheterization in connection with the duration in situ. Twelve catheters removed in under 48 h were bacteriologically negative. Of 42 catheters left in situ for over 48 h, 22 showed positive cultures. This difference was statistically significant ($p < 0.01$). These authors observed an increase of virulence of S. albus due to the intravasal foreign body. Here, too, contamination with hemolytic S. aureus predominated, followed by Proteus, Pseudomonas, Coli, subtilis, Klebsiella, and S. albus. The duration-dependent frequency of bacterial contamination of in-

travasal foreign bodies was confirmed by
SIEWERT (427) who showed infection of
catheters introduced by venesection in
12% when in situ for 1–3 days but in
45% after 3 weeks. Here again hemolytic
S. aureus predominated, followed in this
case by S. albus. MÜLLER (347) on the
other hand found no connection between
infection rate and duration in situ whereas
in our prospective study this was clearly
demonstrable. While our catheter study
was in progress, including bacteriologic
examinations of catheter tip, skin, and
catheter rinsing fluid, BANKS and co-
workers (27) carried out bacteriologic examinations of skin, catheter, and blood
specimens from the catheter vein. They
found, e.g. Staphylococci in 17 skin
swabs, 13 simultaneous catheter swabs,
and in two skin, catheter, and blood cultures. In ten patients both skin and catheter cultures were positive, in two patients
skin, catheter, and blood cultures. Of the
total of 118 catheter examinations 58
proved contaminated.

High rates of bacteremia and septic conditions are reported by ASHCRAFT (12),
COLLINS (107), DILLON (128), DUMA
(137), GLOVER (190), HASSALL (212),
SMITS (432), VUORINEN (473), and WORMS
(491).

In our prospective study (BURRI and GAS-
SER, 88) it was shown that impaired general condition and certain preexisting conditions like diabetes and uremia favor infection on the caval catheter. In
tracheotomized or intubated patients, too,
massive increases of positive bacteriologic
findings were seen, also in hypovolemic or
infectious shock. With preexisting skin
changes the risk of caval catheterization
increases. Venesection caused skin infections in 13.5%, puncture in only 1.4%.
Preexisting thrombosis, phlebitis, or
traumatic injuries in the area of entry or
along the catheter vein affected the infection rate to a high degree. Repeated
puncture attempts increase the danger of
infection. According to our observations

a definite connection is demonstrable between infection and duration in situ. With
increasing duration in situ there are more
frequent skin irritations, skin infections,
inflammations along the catheter vein,
and positive bacteriologic cultures of
swabs from catheter tip, skin, and catheter
rinsing fluid.

Various authors have been concerned
with the prophylaxis of catheter infection.
CHENEY and LINCOLN (99) tested the effect on 135 patients of a 3% tetracycline
ointment applied on the point of entry after introduction of the catheter. They
found no significant reduction of the infection rate after one application of the
antibiotic ointment. It is interesting, however, that with this procedure the infection rate after 24 h remained independent
of the duration. MORAN (344) used
neomycin-bacitracin-polymyxin ointment
and compared it with a placebo. Using the
placebo, infection occurred in 98% of
cases, with the antibiotic ointment only in
18%. Three of the patients treated with
the placebo showed clinical signs of sepsis.
With the use of a broad-spectrum antibiotic such sequelae did not occur. HORIS=
BERGER (242, 243) examined the effect on
the infection rate of a special technical
procedure in introducing the catheter.
One-hundred and thirty-five Intracath
catheters were introduced without any
special precautions. Signs of infection developed in 20 cases, bacteremia in 1, and
confirmed sepsis in 1. If the catheters
were introduced under aseptic precautions
(mask and sterile gloves) the infection
rate was reduced fourfold. These observations are confirmed in a study by BOLASNY
(58) who was able to lower the frequency
of positive catheter cultures by greater attention during introduction from 13% to
4%, that of thrombophlebitis from 12%
to 6% and septic complications from 2%
to 0%. In an examination of 500 catheter
cases FUCHS (178) found positive bac-
teriology in only 3.8%. This low figure is
attributed to the availability of a special

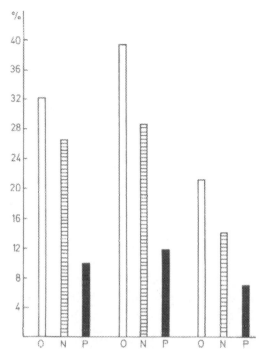

Fig. 40. Infection rate in relation to catheter care

catheter team at the clinic and regular immediate removal of the catheter at the first sign of dysfunction. In our prospective study (BURRI and GASSER 88) we examined the effect of catheter care on the infection rate and found a significant reduction by a daily change of dressings and especially by the use of Polybactrin spray (P) (Fig. 40). In addition, in thrombosis prophylaxis as in the prevention of infectious consequences, the catheter material is of crucial importance since a combination of thrombosis and infection is common.

In view of our latest experiences we are of the opinion that for catheter care a disinfectant solution can be used as effectively as the antibiotic spray. The site of entry of the catheter should be examined daily and sterile dressings renewed.

Vessel Perforations by the Caval Catheter

Vessels can be perforated when the catheter is introduced either during the puncture or by the advancing catheter tip. If the vein is perforated during puncture, at the worst a hematoma develops in the elbow, the leg, or the neck (basilic, femoral, external jugular vein). This represents no great complication, but may make further attempts at puncture impossible. With perforations of the subclavian vein injuries of the pleura, the brachial plexus, and the subclavian artery may occur. Figure 31 shows a hydrothorax due to perforation of the pleura with the catheter in situ. Such sequelae are not merely a hazard with this approach but have been described fairly often. Vessel perforations during puncture are thus of clinical importance practically only with the subclavian vein and anonymous vein.

Vessel wall injuries and perforations during pushing forward of the catheter may occur with any approach. ASHRAF (13), JOHNSON (263), MAHAFFEY (323), GOYANES (197), and BURRI (88) described injuries during introduction of the catheter from the arm, SCHWEIKERT (423) from the external jugular vein, DEUBZNER (124) and EISTERER (146) from the subclavian vein. The consequences of vessel perforation by the catheter tip do not depend on the site of approach. If the injury is situated outside the thoracic region, as in the cases of BURRI (88) and GOYANES (197), a local hematoma develops or, if infusions are administered through the catheter, some tissue change due to the fluid. If the perforation occurs in the region of the subclavian, brachiocephalic, or caval vein, the catheter tip enters the pleural cavity or the mediastinum. In these cases blood transfusion leads to an iatrogenic hemothorax, infusion solution to a hydrothorax (Fig. 31).

Such cases have also been described by ASHRAF (13), SCHWEIKERT (423), DEUBZNER (124), and MAHAFFEY (323). SCHWEIKERT's two cases are unusual insofar as the complications developed in children after only 2 days, possibly due to pressure necrosis of the vessel wall caused by the catheter tip.

The use of soft caval catheters is therefore forced on us to prevent this complication too. A particularly rare observation was described by EISTERER (146) in whose patient the subclavian puncture needle entered the lung and the bronchial tree so that the infusion went into the lung. Immediate removal of the needle and endotracheal suction saved the situation. In the other cases of intrapleural infusion the stoppage of administration together with pleural puncture allowed the patients to recover. Only one patient of DEUBZNER's (124) with an infusion of over 3000 ml into the pleural cavity died of the consequences of this complication, one of FASSOLT's (152) died of his basic disease. Other cases have been described by GALBERT (180), LOERS (313), OTTENI (369), REFETOFF (391), and ROYAL (402). *Altogether we found 41 cases of vessel perforations in the literature, 9 of which ended fatally.*

Cardiac Perforations With Caval Catheter

In rare cases the catheter tip may perforate the right atrium or right ventricle. *We found 41 cases in the available literature; 34 patients died of this complication:* ADAR (1), BRANDT (69), BROWN (76), BURRI (88), CREMER (113), DOERING (130), FITTS (166), FRIEDMANN (176), HENNEBERG (224), McHENRY (225), HENZEL (227), HOMESLEY (241), JOHNSON (263), KLINE (276), KUIPER (288), LOHMÖLLER (317), SCEBAT (408), THOMAS (455), etc. Cardiac perforation by an advancing catheter tip therefore represents a complication extremely dangerous to life and rarely amenable even to immediate active surgery.

Both vascular and cardiac perforations can be largely prevented by cautious technique during introduction of the catheter. *An additional safeguard appears to be the use of a soft catheter material such as polyethylene.* In our opinion the catheter tip must lie in the superior caval vein and must not enter the right atrium or ventricle.

Air Embolism With Caval Catheterization

Much has been written about the possibility of air embolism with caval catheterization but only 24 cases can be found in the literature: BARTH (31), BURRI (88), CRAIG (111), FERRER (158), FLANAGAN (167, 168), GREEN (200), LEVINSKY (308), LUCAS (320). The great majority of these occurred during puncture of the subclavian vein and in four patients this complication caused death.

Air embolism during introduction of a caval catheter through the subclavian, external jugular, or internal jugular vein can be prevented by correct positioning of the patient (Trendelenburg). In patients allowed to walk about with the caval catheter in situ one must ensure a secure connection between the infusion tube and the catheter attachment.

Caval Catheter Embolism

One of the gravest complications of caval catheterization can be embolism of a catheter fragment or of an entire catheter in the central venous circulation. The first report of catheter embolism came from TURNER and SOMMERS (464) in 1954. In 1968 WELLMANN (483) reported 37 cases in the first collective statistics of world literature, 13 of them fatal. With increasing use of caval catheterization the number of reported catheter embolisms rose rapidly: AL-ABRAK (6), APFELBERG (8), AYERS (20), BARRY (32), BERNHARDT (47), BERTHO (48), BETT (49), BLAIR (50), BLOOS (55), DE BOARD (56), BORGESKOV (60), BURRI (88), CARNEY (95), CHODKIEWICZ (100), COBLENTZ (103), DICKERSON (126), DOERING (130), EDWARDS (143, 144), FUNKE (177), GOTTSCHALL (195), HERBERT (228), HOLDER (239), HUTH (249), KESSLER (273), KLÖTZER (277), KLUGE (278), KNUTSON (279, 280),

Kux (290), Lamprecht (292, 293), Mariano (326), Mathey (330), Mühe (346), Nash (353), Nissen-Druey (356), Northcutt (359), Pässler (374, 375), Porstmann (381), McRae (384), Richardson (393), Ross (398), Steinert (440), Taylor (450, 451), Thomas (456), Tsingoglou (461), Tulgan (463), Turner (464), Udwadia (465), v. Ungern (466), and Wellmann (482, 483).

So far we have collected and evaluated 315 cases of catheter embolism in the venous system: 254 cases we found in the literature, mainly case reports, and 44 cases were discovered by written inquiry from 45 clinics and institutions in German-speaking countries. Fourteen cases were seen in our own clinics and 3 occurred during a prospective study with 3241 caval catheterizations (88).

The fact that the inquiry produced at least one catheter embolism from nearly every clinic by itself suggests a hidden incidence of such events which may amount to a multiple of the known cases. We estimate the *incidence* of catheter embolism as 0.1% on the basis of the prospective study.

The *reason* for introducing a caval catheter was accident in 17.3% (average age of this group 30.7 years), surgical operation or emergency operation in 27.2% (aver-

age age 50.4 years), and medical (nonsurgical) indication in 46.1% (average age 44.5 years). In 9.4% of cases the catheter embolism occurred through separation of part of the tube in hydrocephalus drainage (average age 6.4 years).

The *age distribution* of catheter embolism is shown in Figure 41, with higher incidence emerging in the fifth to eighth decade.

Mechanism of Catheter Embolism

In 118 cases we found either vague data or none at all. In one-half — exactly 49% — of the remaining 196 catheter embolisms cutting off of the catheter at the point of the needle was given as the cause

Table 13

Mechanism of catheter embolism	n	%
Catheter		
severed by needle	96	49,0
broken off	30	15,3
torn off	23	11,7
separated	25	12,8
"disappeared"	22	11,2
Total	196	100,0
No data	118	

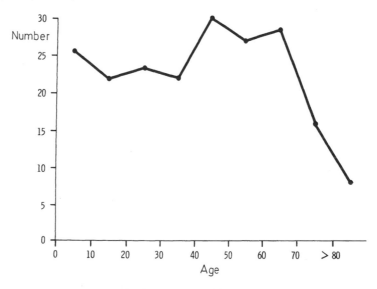

Fig. 41. Age distribution of caval catheter embolism

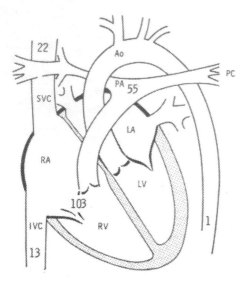

Fig. 42. Localization of catheter fragment emboli

Table 14

Site of approach	n	%
Arm vein	73	52,5
Femoral vein	13	9,4
Saphenous vein	3	2,2
Pudendal vein	1	0,7
Peripheral total	90	64,7
External jugular vein	6	4,3
Internal jugular vein	1	0,7
Subclavian vein	42	35,2
Near-heart total	49	35,3
Total	139	100,0

Table 15

Localization of catheter embolism	n
Peripheral	70
Central	225
Paradoxical	1
Unknown or no data	19
Total	315

of embolism (Table 13). Other causes were far less frequent: broken off in 15.3%, torn off in 11.7%, separated in 12.8%, and disappeared unnoticed for no ascertainable cause in 11.2%.

Catheter Embolism in Relation to Site of Approach

A detailed summary is given in Table 14 which shows that mostly (64.7%) peripheral veins had been chosen for the approach. In 70 cases the catheter fragment came to rest peripherally and could be removed by a minor operation (Table 15). In 225 cases, however, the fragment was washed away into the central system. In 32 of these cases no particulars on the central localization were given. The distribution of cases with known localization is shown in Figure 42. Most frequently, i. e., in 103 cases, the fragment was found in the right heart. In another case the fragment reached the arterial system via a patent oval foramen. It was found at autopsy as an incidental finding in a renal artery. In 19 cases localization was impossible because the catheters were not radio-opaque or adequate data were absent (Table 15).

Figure 43 shows a case of catheter embolism where during intensive therapy two catheter fragments formed emboli. A piece of 5 cm was in a right pulmonary artery and one of 20 cm in the right atrium and right ventricle. Other examples are shown in Figures 44 and 45.

Consequences Depending on Site of Embolism (Table 16)

Only in 5 out of the 315 cases evaluated did we find no indication as to how the catheter fragment was removed or whether it was left alone. In 3 of these cases the embolism was peripheral. Out of 70 embolisms of peripheral localization, 61 were removed surgically, 59 of them by direct operation (exposure) and 2 transvenously. In 3 other cases no data

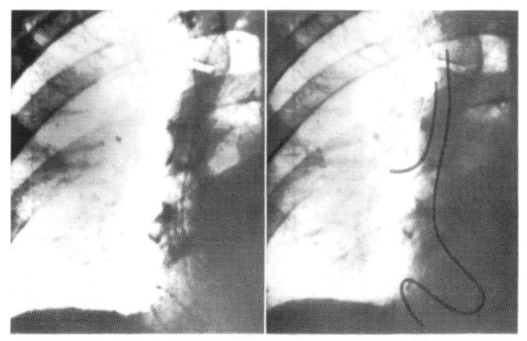

Fig. 43. Double catheter embolism. Original picture, showing catheter fragments

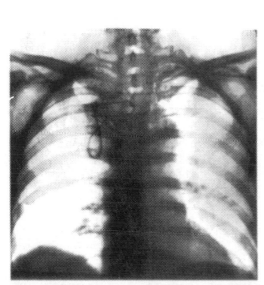

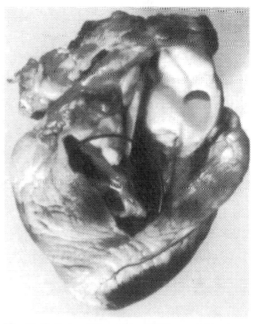

Fig. 44. Seldinger spiral embolus in subclavian, anonymous, and superior caval vein

Fig. 45. Catheter fragment in right heart (sheep)

Table 16

Localization of embolism	n Left alone	n Of which died
Caval vein	10	2 = 20,0%
Right heart	28	15 = 53,6%
Pulmonary artery	11	1 = 9,1%
Renal artery	1	0
"Central"	6	0
Central total	56	18 = 32,1%
Unknown	19	2 = 10,5%
Total	75	20 = 26,7%

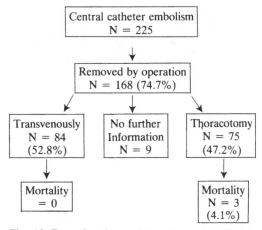

Fig. 46. Fate of patients with catheter embolism in relation to therapeutic measures

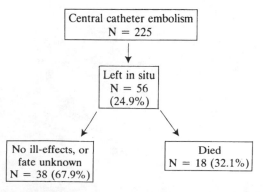

Fig. 47. Mortality after catheter emboli left in situ

of the type of operation were given. Six catheter fragments were left alone and during the period of observation no death in connection with this occurred.

Two-hundred and twenty-five catheter fragments formed emboli in the central venous system, another in a renal artery by way of a patent oval foramen. Of the 225 central emboli, 168 (74.7%) were removed surgically (Fig. 46), 84 (52.8%) of these by an indirect transvenous method without any fatal complications and 75 (47.2%) by operation, mostly thoracotomy and cardiotomy. Three patients died following thoracotomy, a mortality of 4.1%.

Eighteen patients (32.1%) died of consequences of catheter fragments left alone (Fig. 47). Analyzed according to the localization of the central embolism (Table 16), the mortality in this group of fragments left in the right heart was as high as 53.6%. Localization in a pulmonary artery seemed to be tolerated better, with a mortality of only 9.1%.

Catheter-Induced Causes of Death

There were altogether 20 confirmed catheter-induced deaths due to non-removal of the emboli. The most frequent cause of death was perforation of the cardiac wall (5 times), in 3 cases it was septic endocarditis, in 3 others therapy-resistant arrhythmia with cardiac failure, in 3 cases caval thrombosis and pulmonary embolism, in 2 cases cardiac wall necrosis, in 1 case sepsis and in 1 case caval thrombosis with pericarditis. In the 19 cases with unknown localization of the embolus the cause of death was always septic thrombophlebitis.

Extraction of Catheter Emboli

Various procedures for the removal of catheter emboli are reported by numerous authors: BANKS (28), BARMAN (30), BASHOUR (33), BEAULIEU (38), BLOCK

(53), BLOOMFIELD (54), DELANY (123), DOTTER (133), EDELSTEIN (141), FISHER (165), GARCIA (182), GERACI (188), GSCHNITZER (204), HAMMERMEISTER (211), HELMER (218, 219), HENLEY (222), HIPONA (236), HODEL (237), HUTH (249), HYMAN (250), IRMER (252), LETH (307), LILLEHEI (310), LOERS (316), MARKKULA (327), MARLON (328), MASSUMI (329), MATHUR (332), MAUTHE (334), MILLER (341), MIRHOSEINI (342), PORSTMANN (381), RANNINGER (387), RASHKIND (389), ROSSI (401), SCHECHTER (413), SHANDER (424), SMITHWICK (431), SMYTH (433), SONI (435), MCSWEENEY (447), TATSUMI (449), TRUSLER (460), VAUGHN (468).

Transvenous Extraction of Catheter
(Table 17)

Since MASSUMI (329) succeeded for the first time in 1967 in successfully removing a catheter piece washed into the caval vein indirectly with the aid of a catheter and a fine wire loop, the relatively major operation of thoracotomy has been increasingly abandoned in favor of various indirect transvenous methods. A survey of the different extraction instruments now in use is shown in Table 17. It proved

possible with their aid to remove from the caval vein catheter pieces washed into the central system in 73.9%, from the right heart in 60% and even from the pulmonary arteries in 38.6%.

1. Loop Technique

Fragments were removed most frequently with loop-carrying catheters. These were either terminal loops with a double-running elastic wire or synthetic thread or terminal or lateral loops with a single-running wire, similar to the Zeiss loop also in use (Fig. 48). Of 84 catheter fragments, 43 (51.2%) were removed in this way, 13

Table 17

	Caval vein & rt. heart	Pulmonary artery	Alltogether
Loop	30	13	43 (51,2%)
Endoscopy forceps	16	0	16 (19,0%)
"Hooked catheter"	9	0	9 (10,7%)
Ureteric stone extractor	7	1	8 (9,5%)
Catheter grasping forceps	3	0	3 (3,6%)
No data	5	0	5 (6,0%)
Total	70	14	84 (100,0%)

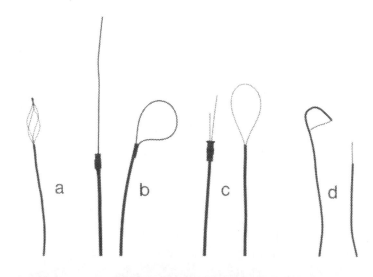

Fig. 48. Different loops for transvenous extraction of catheter emboli

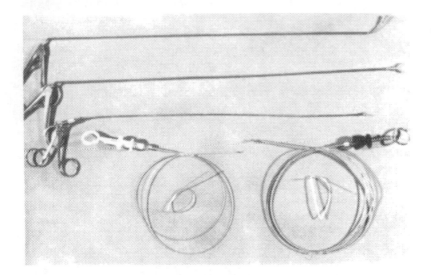

Fig. 49. Forceps for transvenous extraction of catheter emboli

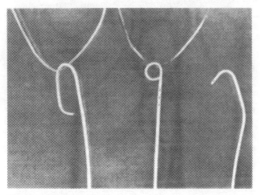

Fig. 50. Hooked instruments. *Left:* coronary catheter according to *Judkins. Centre:* "pigtail" catheter. *Right:* coronary catheter according to *Sones*

via the jugular vein, also flexible bladder biopsy forceps, stomach biopsy forceps, and myocardium biopsy forceps. These instruments, however, have definite drawbacks.

1. They are relatively or absolutely rigid and there is therefore a danger of venous wall perforation.
2. The forceps may produce serious intima or endocardial lesions.

In our opinion their use should therefore be dispensed with. Only PORSTMANN (381) developed a forceps specially for intravenously dislodged foreign bodies which seems to be less dangerous owing to its spirally rounded ends.

of them from the pulmonary arteries. It is undoubtedly a very simple, yet effective and safe method. Such a suitable instrument can be produced anywhere in emergencies without any trouble.

2. Endoscopy Forceps

Endoscopy forceps of various kinds (Fig. 49) were used successfully in 16 cases or 19.0%. Among them there were even rigid bronchoscopy forceps, introduced

3. Hooked Catheters

Hooked catheters as used in various forms in angiography (Fig. 50) were successfully used in nine cases. The bent tip of this catheter can be straightened with a mandrin (tip deflector guide) so that sticking at the tricuspid valve or at a papillary muscle and injury to the venous wall or endocardium are preventable. This sticking was observed with rigid, hooked catheters previously in use and necessitated thoracotomy or cardiotomy.

4. Ureteric Stone Extractor

Instruments whose basket-like loop unfolds sufficiently and which are sufficiently flexible, as the Dormia stone extractor shown in Fig. 48, were used in seven cases without causing any harm. DOTTER (133) suggested a ureteric stone extractor modified by him for this purpose. Similar in principle is the instrument specially developed experimentally by RANNINGER (387) for the removal of foreign body emboli. However, no reports on its clinical use have been published so far.

5. Fogarty Catheter

This may be useful for fragments whose central end has not yet reached the atrium, especially in peripheral catheter embolism (MARLON, 328; MATHUR, 332).

Chances of Success With Indirect Methods

There are few data available in the evaluated literature on failures of transvenous extraction of catheters washed into the central veins. It emerges from Table 18 that the transvenous attempt had to be abandoned in 11 cases. In 3 cases the catheter fragment was in the caval vein, in another 3 cases in the right heart and in 5 cases in the pulmonary artery. Five fragments were left alone and the patients had no symptoms as far as is known. In 6 cases they were removed by thoracotomy.

Table 18

	Unsuccessful	Left alone	Thoracotomy
Caval vein	3	2	1
Right heart	3	2	1
Pulmonary artery	5	1	4
Total	11	5	6

In 6 reported cases several attempts were required for successful extraction, mostly with different instruments. Only a few authors gave particulars of difficulties and incidents during transvenous extraction but they are probably far more frequent than this figure suggests.

An apparently rare complication is the breaking off of catheter parts during extraction. Only HUTH (249) reported in 1973 that this happened in three out of four catheter embolisms observed by him. In two cases an attempt was made to remove a catheter washed into the right heart by thoracotomy and cardiotomy with a forceps when parts broke off on grasping the catheter and were washed into the pulmonary artery, as shown by a postoperative thorax radiograph. In another case it was possible to grasp the catheter transvenously with a loop but here again a 5-cm-long piece broke off and was later found in a pulmonary artery. In all cases the quality of catheter material was said to be poor. It is known of PVC catheters left in the circulation for a long period that the material becomes hard and brittle due to the disappearance of the softeners.

Deaths did not occur with the use of indirect methods, 56 cases so far. Transvenous removal therefore now seems possible without significant risk even with poor general condition.

Conclusions

In 1970 BENEDICT (40) still maintained that that "to try to remove broken-off pieces of catheter was more traumatic and more dangerous than to leave the harmless catheters alone." He himself had seen at least eight cases where the catheter was left alone and caused no serious complications. The aforementioned reports and the result of this study however show the danger of leaving catheter fragments alone and the often deleterious consequences. Last but not least it should be pointed out that in 1968 in the USA the Washington Supreme Court decided that the hospital concerned and the personnel responsible were liable for a catheter embolism and its consequences.

It is therefore necessary to take measures to prevent catheter embolism at all costs but if it does occur, prompt action is required:

1. In case of catheter embolism radiologic and, if necessary, angiographic localization and subsequent surgical extraction must be demanded. Sometimes it is possible to prevent the catheter from being washed into the central veins by proximal compression. In any case transvenous removal with a suitable instrument (e. g., loop) should be tried first before considering thoracotomy. Exclusive use of radio-opaque catheters is a precondition.

2. Far more important, we believe, are meaningful measures for the prevention of this complication. Its causes suggest the following guidelines:

1. The site of entry of the catheter or the needle tip should not be directly over a joint and must be fixed. In restless patients the extremity must be immobilized.

2. The catheter must not be retracted through the needle either during introduction or for correction. Obstacles should be overcome by changing the position of the head or arm or by starting the infusion early. If this does not succeed, the needle must be removed with the tube and the puncture repeated elsewhere.

3. Only catheter models with removable metal or plastic needles should be used to exclude cutting off.

Rarest Complications of Caval Catheterization

An extremely rare consequence of subclavian puncture, to recognise the possibility of which, however, is absolutely indispensable, is injury to the brachial plexus. We found four such cases in the literature; two of them recovered, in the two others a permanent lesion remained.

YAROM (493) stated in 1964 that tracheal injuries during subclavian puncture in small children would occur relatively often. KÖSTERS (282) described a perforation of a struma follicle during the same approach. BRENNAN (70) saw a venotracheal fistula after catheterization, BLITT (52) saw a puncture of the cuff of a tracheal tube and LARSEN (299) an injury to the internal mammary artery.

Immediately following a subclavian puncture under local anesthesia OBEL (361) saw a temporary phrenic paresis due to the action of the local anesthetic on the nerve. PARIKH (376) described the development of Horner's syndrome after puncture of the internal jugular vein.

Probably the most unusual complication of caval catheterization was reported by GOYANES (197). In a patient with a major soft tissu operation on the shoulder girdle the nurse mistook the caval catheter for the polyvinyl tube of the redon drain. The blood transfusion therefore went into the fresh operation wound while the redon bottle filled up with blood from the patient's vein. The patient's condition deteriorated but the mistake was discovered soon enough to prevent a fatal conclusion.

VIII. Frequent Autopsy Findings in Patients With Caval Catheters

In the autoptic evaluation of anatomic findings in patients with caval catheters we are struck by complicating conditions that must be regarded as consequences of catheterization. They are mainly sequelae of thrombosis and infection. Relatively harmless are the very common precipitation thromboses which envelop the catheter (Fig. 51), more rarely one finds thrombotic changes on the tricuspid valve and on the tip of the cavel catheter in the region of the right ventricle. These two localizations indicate the dangers of wrong catheter positions in the heart. The pathogenesis of this thrombus formation is still largely uncertain. We have learned in atherosclerosis that collagen released in the area of an atheromatous ulcer causes aggregation of the platelets, whereby ADP is liberated from the aggregated thrombocytes and again causes more platelets to aggregate. The same phenomena are demonstrable in animal experiments when the endothelial layer of the intima is injured. Here, too, there is platelet aggregation under the action of collagen, not uncommonly leading to parietal thrombosis. The exploration of the collagen molecules and the discovery of the amino acid, glucine, of hydroxyproline and glucosized hydroxylysin in the collagen molecules led to a discussion on the participation of a complement factor in the development of thrombosis. It was found that a part of the first complement component, namely C_1q, also a glucine, contains hydroxylysin. Since contamination with bacterial substrates may occur during introduction of catheter into the caval vein, there is quite a possibility of bacterial substrate entering into a reaction with this part of the first complement component in some still unexplained manner, whereby complement, instead of col-

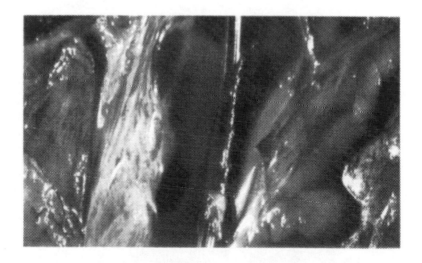

Fig. 51. Ensheathing thrombi on catheter

lagen molecules, would cause coagulation by aggregation of thrombocytes. Catheter material may also fix C_1q. These speculations are still mostly hypothetic but certainly worth pursuing.

The other common complication of caval catheterization is infection. Besides infection at the entry site of the catheter the pathologist finds bacterial contamination of thrombi around the catheter or on the tricuspid valve (Fig. 52) where opportunistic organismus but also pyogenic organisms like Staphylococci and Streptococci may be demonstrable. These infections occur especially in patients with infections by the same organisms in a locality unconnected with the catheter. This makes it likely that at least some infections of thrombosis originate not by way of the caval catheter but hematogenously, by bacteria settling on the culture medium of thrombi and multiplying.

The fate of such thrombi varies. They may cicatrise and, as it were, heal up, in which case a harmless substrate remains in the form of thickening of the vein. But they may also separate and cause pulmonary embolism. Generally these embolisms are not fatal, owing to the extent of the thrombosis. We know that in man large

and very small thromboembolisms in the lungs are very dangerous whereas those of medium size become dangerous for the patient only if more than 50% of the diameter of the pulmonary arteries is occupied by the embolus. Massive embolism obstructing the main branches of the pulmonary artery leads to right heart failure. Such embolism is rare in patients with catheters because the extent of the thrombosis is insufficient. Microembolisms consisting mainly of platelets may cause death from right heart failure even in small numbers, due to release of peptide-like agents from the thrombocytes leading to bronchospasm with atelectasis and pulmonary hypertension. However, these small emboli, mostly consisting exclusively of platelets, are also rare as sole consequences of thrombosis around the catheter because the caval catheter produces not merely an aggregation of platelets but true parietal thromboses. In the great majority of cases the microembolisms of platelet aggregates in the lungs are due to resuscitation of the peripheral circulation paralyzed by shock where microthrombi had formed.

That leaves the medium-sized embolisms, of which it may be said that the extent or

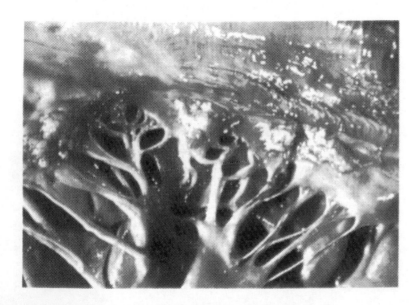

Fig. 52. Septic infective endocarditis of mitral valve with subclavian catheter

quantity of parietal or ensheathing thromboses in patients with caval catheters is mostly in sufficient to obstruct more than 50% of the pulmonary arteries. When such embolisms are found at autopsy, the pathologist mostly hears nothing about the patient's symptoms, and death is attributed to some cause other than embolism. In preexisting left heart insufficiency with pulmonary congestion an infarct (Fig. 53) develops in the supply area of the vessel blocked by embolism, with infarct pleurisy which clinically arouses attention by pleuritic pains.

The clinical picture of embolism changes decisively if the thrombi are contaminated with bacteria. Here even medium-sized pulmonary embolisms lead to septic-hemorrhagic infarction and hematogenous abscesses (Fig. 54) which then lead to

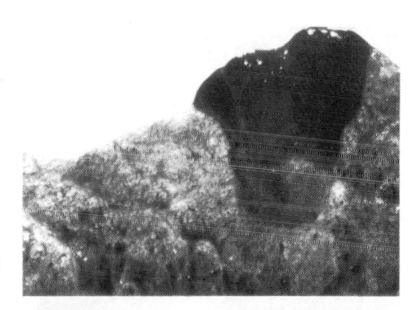

Fig. 53. Fresh hemorrhagic infarct in patient with caval catheter and coexisting congestion

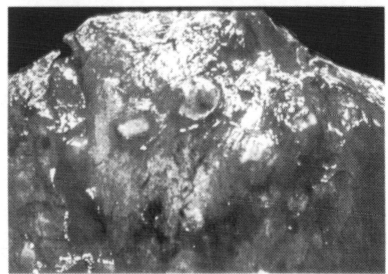

Fig. 54. Multiple septic lung abscesses and purulent septic lung infarcts in patient with caval catheter (catheter sepsis)

hematogenous pneumonia. The statement that in the lung only the large and multiple small embolisms consisting mainly of platelets are dangerous to life does not apply to these bacterially contaminated thromboembolisms. Medium-sized embolisms entering different pulmonary branches may also cause death from sepsis and septicopyemia due to purulent infarction.

In the experience of pathologists, all other consequences of caval catheterization are numerically of no importance. In acute deaths after introduction of a caval catheter the autopsy must be carried out suspecting air embolism. The same caution is required for conducting an autopsy if there is a suspicion of catheter-induced pneumothorax. Hematomas may be found, very rarely torn catheters, wrong catheter positions with or without perforation of the vein, and hemothorax. In the experience of the Ulm pathologists these complications of caval catheterization have not caused any deaths.

IX. Recommendations for Caval Catheterization

On the basis of the available catheter models and technical possibilities, and taking into consideration the complications to be anticipated and their frequency, we make the following recommendations:

1. Indications

a) *Measurement of CVP and Substitution Therapy*
Patient in dangerous circulatory condition (shock, threatening shock)
Preparation for major, risky surgical operation
Surgical operation on a high-risk patient
b) *Parenteral Feeding*
Administration of hypertonic solutions
c) *Lasting Venous Access* (relative)

2. Catheter Material

Siliconized polyethylene
Removable cannula
Certainty of sterile use

3. Approach

a) *Leg Veins*
In view of the high complication rate with thrombosis/embolism, local infection/sepsis, this approach in adults should in our opinion be forbidden.
Exception: if all other approaches are barred by local skin changes (e. g., burns).
b) *Arm Veins*
Puncture of the basilic vein is simple but pushing the catheter forward relatively often proves difficult. The absence of puncture-induced complications makes this approach advisable for beginners. Late complications such as thrombosis and infection are common but their rate can be reduced by careful observation and care of the catheter entry site during the whole period the catheter is in situ.
c) *Subclavian Vein*
Aubaniac's technique is clearly superior to Yoffa's and to puncture of the anonymous vein. The dangers of this approach lie in the puncture itself when the artery or plexus but above all the pleura may be injured. The puncture must be carried out only by an expert or in the presence of one. In patients with preexisting pulmonary or cardiac lesions we recommend that subclavian puncture be avoided.
d) *External Jugular Vein*
Puncture and introduction of the catheter very often prove dificult but the complications are harmless and rare. The approach by the external jugular vein should therefore be considered only if the vessel is clearly demonstrable, takes a straight course and if sufficient time is available. The external jugular vein must for the present be considered as a "reserve approach."
e) *Internal Jugular Vein*
The difficulty of internal jugular puncture is the same as that of subclavian puncture. The need for an expert therefore applies to this approach as well. The certainty of correct placement of the catheter tip after successful puncture — expecially with the right-sided approach — and the extremely low complication rate make the internal

jugular puncture under clinical conditions the approach of choice.

General

The approaches to the caval vein by the subclavian and internal jugular vein are reserved for the expert.
The inexperienced should keep to the basilic or external jugular vein.
Previously damaged tissue (previous puncture attempts, irritation, thrombosis, infection, burns) should be avoided for approaches to the caval vein.

4. Technical Procedure

a) Puncture, not venesection
b) Peripheral catheter in situ for a maximum of 48 h
c) Degreasing and careful disinfection of a wide area of skin around the puncture site
d) Local anesthesia in conscious patients is recommended for subclavian and internal jugular puncture
e) For these approaches sterile coverage is required
f) Atraumatic puncture.
   Catheter model with sharp-ground needle, avoidance of repeated puncture attempts in the same place
g) The use of sterile gloves, cap, and mask is recommended if sufficient time is available. It is obligatory if further manipulations are required during introduction.
h) Careful pushing forward of the catheter without the use of force.
i) Difficulties in pushing the catheter forward can mostly be removed by injection of normal saline solution or starting the infusion early, together with changing the position of the body or pulling and rotating the arm. In such situations sterile coverings should be used and the surgeon should wear sterile gloves.

k) Radiologic control of the catheter tip
   Screening while pushing the catheter forward
   standard radiograph of thorax
   if uncertain, injection of contrast medium
l) Correct catheter position means the superior caval vein, not the right atrium or ventricle (perforation, damage due to pressure). Wrong catheter position demands immediate correction and repeated control.
m) No retraction of the catheter through the needle in situ (catheter embolism)
n) Careful fixation of catheter tube (possibly sewing on)

5. Care of Catheter

a) Entry site to be examined daily:
   Application of disinfectant or Polybactrin spray
   Sterile covering or open treatment
   No dressing sprays (retention)
b) Daily rinsing of catheter with normal saline and after each transfusion or blood withdrawal
c) Change of infusion set after each infusion but at least daily
d) Sterile handling of the connection between caval catheter and infusion set and of the infusion
e) Secure connection between caval catheter and infusion set (air embolism)

6. Removal of Caval Catheter

a) As soon as no longer absolutely necessary
b) With irritation or inflammation of catheter entry site
c) With irritation or inflammation of catheter-carrying vein
d) With pains
e) With fever of uncertain origin (swab of catheter tip after removal, blood culture)
f) With signs of thrombosis (swelling)

7. General

a) No prophylactic general administration of antibiotics for caval catheterization
b) No general administration of anticoagulants for caval catheterization.

8. Special Guidelines

a) Caval Catheterization at the Place of Emergency
– In dangerous emergencies a puncture of peripheral veins with self-retaining needles should be tried if it seems likely to succeed in view of the filling state of the vein, since serious complications need not be anticipated.
– Puncture of central veins for caval catheterization under emergency conditions should be performed only by a surgeon who has learned the procedure under nonemergency hospital conditions.
– In emergency situations we recommend for the expert first subclavian puncture, next internal jugular puncture.
– If a little more time is available, puncture of the internal jugular vein may be attempted even in emergencies because of the lower complication rate.
– In states of severe collapse those with little experience in the puncture of central veins should try puncture and, if necessary, short-distance cannulation of the external jugular vein if adequately filled.
– In traumatization of the thoracic area

that side should – paradoxically – be chosen for central puncture on which a hemothorax or pneumothorax is suspected. By this procedure additional impairment of the respiratory system by puncture complications is avoided.

b) Caval Catheter in Children
– The femoral and unbilical veins are not suitable approaches for a caval catheter.
– Punctures of the basilic and external jugular vein pose certain problems but should always be used primarily by those with no experience in other methods.
– The approach to the caval vein by the internal jugular and subclavian vein should be taken only with sufficient experience.
An exception is in acute emergencies where only the subclavian approach often promises success.
N.B.: Local infections become generalized much more quickly in children than in adults. Careful management is essential.

c) Exposure of Vein
Indication: if puncture is not (any longer) possible.
Performance:
– Strictest surgical asepsis
– No ligation of catheter-carrying vein
– Removal of catheter through separate skin incision
– Nursing as with caval catheter after puncture

References

1. Adar, R., Mozes, M.: Fatal complications of central venous catheters. Br Med J **1971/III**, 746.
2. Ahnefeld, F. W., Burri, C., Dick, W., Halmágyi, M.: Infusionstherapie II, Parenterale Ernährung. Klin. Anaesth. u. Intensivtherapie Vol. 7 Berlin-Heidelberg-New York: Springer 1975.
3. Ahnefeld, F. W., Gorgass, B., Dick, W.: Organisatorische und medizinische Probleme bei der vorklinischen Versorgung von Polytraumatisierten. Notfallmedizin **2**, 166 (1976).
4. Allgöwer, M.: Mesures diagnostiques dans l'appréciation des traumatisés graves. Méd Hyg **23**, 503 (1965).
5. Allgöwer, M., Gruber, U. F.: Schockpathogenese und ihre Differentialdiagnose. Chirurg **38**, 97 (1967).
6. Al-Abrak, M., Samuel, J. R.: An unusual case of breaking of a central venous catheter. Anaesthesia **29**, 585 (1974).
7. Altmann, R. P., Randolph, J. G.: Application and hazards of total parenteral nutrition in infants. Ann Surg **174**, 85 (1971).
8. Apfelberg, D. B., Bernie, J., Johnson, W. D., Watson, R., Lepley, D.: Polyethylene catheter embolization to the heart. Wis Med J **67**, 108, (1969).
9. Apoil, A., Pintoux, D.: Accidents des cathéters intraveineux. Ann Chir **25**, 507 (1971).
10. Arnold, S., Feathers, R. S., Gibbs, E.: Bilateral pneumothoraxes and subcutaneous emphysema, a complication of internal jugular venepuncture. Br Med J 1973/I, 211.
11. Ashbough, D., Thomson, J. W.: Subclavian-vein infusion. Lancet 1963/II, 1138.
12. Ashcraft, K. W., Leape, L. L.: Candida sepsis complicating parenteral feeding. JAMA **212**, 454 (1972).
13. Ashraf, M. M.: Venous perforation due to polyethylene catheter. Ann Surg **157**, 375 (1963).
14. Atik, M.: Application and proper interpretation of central venous pressure monitoring in the management of shock. Ann Surg **33**, 118 (1967).
15. Aubaniac, R.: Une nouvelle voie d'injection ou de ponction veineuse. Sem Hôp Paris **28**, 3445 (1952).
16. Aubaniac, R.: L'injection intraveineuse sousclaviculaire. Presse Méd **60**, 1456 (1952).
17. Aubaniac, R.: L'angio-cardiographie par voie sousclaviculaire. Presse Méd **62**, 1308 (1954).
18. Aubaniac, R.: La voie sous-claviculaire. Rev Prat **2**, 65 (1959).
19. Aulenbacher, C. E.: Hydrothorax from subclavian veincatheterization. JAMA **214**, 372 (1970).
20. Ayers, W. B.: Fatal intracardiac embolization from indwelling intravenous polyethylene catheter. Arch Surg **75**, 259 (1957).
21. Bach, H. G., Slowinski, St., Rummel, H., Kuhn, W.: Punktion und Kathetrismus der Vena subclavia. Anaesthesist **16**, 223 (1967).
22. Baden, H.: Perkutan kateterisation of v. subclavia. Nord Med **71**, 590 (1964).
23. Baden, H.: Percutaneous subclavian-vein catheterization complicated by infusion into the pleural cavity. Nord Med **72**, 1416 (1964).
24. Bär, F.: Die gesundheitliche Beurteilung der Kunststoffe und anderer hochmolekularer Stoffe im Rahmen des Lebensmittelgesetzes. Bundesgesundheitsblatt 5, 9. März 1962.
25. Bässler, R., Reichelt, A.: Die Feinstruktur der Oberfläche von Kunststoffkathetern. Anaesthesiologie und Wiederbelebung Vol. 13, "Infusionstherapie" Berlin-Heidelberg-New York: Springer 1966.
26. Bahn, C. H., Kennedy, M. T.: Catheterization of the superior vena cava. Surgery **73**, 115 (1973).
27. Banks, D. C., Cawdrey, H. M., Harries, M. G., Kidner, P. H., Yales, D. B.: Infection from intravenous catheters. Lancet 1970/I., 1644.
28. Banks, T., Yeoh, H. H.: Removal of embolized catheter. Postgrad Med **51**, 116 (1972).
29. Bansmer, G., Keith, D., Tesluk, H.: Complications following use of indwelling catheters of inferior vena cava. JAMA **167**, 1606 (1958).
30. Barman, P. C., Syracuse, N. Y.: A simple method for removal of polyethylene catheters from the pulmonary artery. J Thorac Cardiovasc Surg **65**, 792 (1973).
31. Barth, L., Richter, J.: Untersuchungen zum Mechanismus der Luftembolie im Bereich der

Halsvenen der Menschen. Anaesthesist **20**, 430 (1971).

32. Barry, W. F., McIntosh, J. R., Whalen, R. E.: A radiographic demonstration of a polyethylene catheter lying free in the superior vena cava. N Engl J Med **267**, 1194 (1962).

33. Bashour, T. T., Banks, T., Cheng, T. O.: Retrieval of lost catheters by a myocardial biopsy catheter device. Chest **66**, 395 (1974).

34. Bauer, H.: Über die Komplikationen des Vena-subclavia-Katheters und deren Verhütung. Infusionstherapie **2**, 134 (1975).

35. Bauer, H.: Gefahren des Vena-subclavia-Katheters. Dtsch Med Wochenschr **101**, 672 (1976).

36. Bauer, U., Hasse, W.: Die Anwendung des Umbilicalvenen- und Vena-cava-Katheters in der Intensivpflege. Z Kinderchir **13**, 2 (1973).

37. Baumann, W., Greinacher, J.: Der Cava-Katheter in der pädiatrischen Intensivpflege. Anaesth Prax **10**, 109, (1975).

38. Beaulieu, M., Gravel, J. A.: Cardiotomie pour ablation d'un cathéter intraveineux. Laval Méd **31**, 458 (1961).

39. Becher, D. P., Nulsen, F. E.: Control of hydrocephalus by valveregulated venous shunt: avoidance of complications in prolonged shunt maintenance. J Neurosurg **28**, 215 (1968).

40. Benedict, J. S.: Provocative words about "guild ridden physicians". Chest **58**, 554 (1970).

41. Bennett, R. J.: Use of intravenous plastic catheters. Br med J **1963/II**, 1236.

42. Bentley, D. W., Lepper, M. H.: Septicaemia related to indwelling venous catheter. JAMA **206**, 1749 (1968).

43. Berger, A., Dinstl, K.: Die chirurgischen Probleme in der Intensivpflegestation. Wien Klin Wochenschr **77**, 962 (1965).

44. Bergmann, J. A., Aaron, R. K.: Subclavian catheters in cardiac arrest. JAMA **217**, 210 (1971).

45. Bernhard, R. W., Stahl, W. M.: Subclavian vein-catheterization: A prospective study. Noninfection complications. Ann Surg **173**, 184 (1971).

46. Bernhard, R. W., Stahl, W. M., Chase, R. M.: Subclavian vein-catheterization: A prospective study. Infections complications. Ann Surg **173**, 191 (1971).

47. Bernhardt, L. C., Wegner, G. P., Mendentiall, J. T.: Intravenous catheter embolization to the pulmonary artery. Chest **57**, 329 (1970).

48. Bertho, E., Ratte, J., Gagnon, J. C.: Etude clinique et expérimentale des cathéters intraveineux embolisés. Union Med Can **99**, 58 (1970).

49. Bett, J. H., Anderson, S. T.: Plastic catheter embolism to the right heart. A technique of nonsurgical removal. Med J Aust **2**, 854 (1971).

50. Blair, E., Hunziker, R., Flanagan, M. E.: Catheter embolism. Surgery **67**, 457 (1970).

51. Bleweff, J. M., Kyger, E. R., Patterson, L. T.: Subclavian vein-catheter replacement without venepuncture. Arch Surg **108**, 241 (1974).

52. Blitt, C. D., Wright, W. A.: An unusual complication of percutaneous internal jugular vein cannulation, puncture of an endotracheal tube cuff. Anaesthesia **40**, 306 (1974).

53. Block, P. C.: Transvenous retrieval of foreign bodies in the cardiac circulation. JAMA **224**, 241 (1973).

54. Bloomfield, D. A.: Techniques of non-surgical retrieval of iatrogenic foreign bodies from the heart. Am J Cardiol **27**, 538 (1971).

55. Bloos, J., Flörkemeier, V., Schmücker, K.: Venenkatheterembolie. Med Welt **23**, 261 (1972).

56. De Board, R. A., Elwood, P., Hart, R.: Removal of pudenz catheter from the heart. J Thorac Cardiovasc Surg **56**, 236 (1968).

57. Boeckmann, C. K., Krill, C. E.: Infections complicating parenteral alimentation in infants and children. J Pediatr Surg **5**, 117 (1970).

58. Bolasny, B. L., Martin, Ch. E., Conkle, D. M.: Careful technique with plastic intravenous catheters. Surg Gynecol Obstet **132**, 1030 (1971).

59. Bonner, C. D.: Experience with plastic tubing in prolonged intravenous therapy. N Engl J Med **245**, 97, (1951).

60. Borgeskov, S., Lauridsen, P., Rugg, I. H.: Iatrogene fremmedlegemer i cor og de store kar. Nord Med **76**, 828 (1966).

61. Borja, A. R., Hinshaw, J. R.: A safe way to perform infraclavicular subclavian vein Catheterization. Surg Gynecol Obstet **130**, 673 (1907).

62. Borja, A. R., Berja, E. R., Ramirez, H.: Deaths from subclavian vein-catheterization. Chest **60**, 517 (1971).

63. Bork, F.: Linksseitiger Infusionshydrothorax infolge eines Dauerkatheterismus der oberen Hohlvene. Dtsch Gesundheitsw **27**, 937 (1972).

64. Borow, M.: The use of central venous pressure as an accurate guide for body fluid replacement. Surg Gynecol Obstet **3**, 545 (1965).

65. Borst, H. G.: Neuzeitliche Schocktherapie. Chirurg **38**, 104 (1967).

66. Boruchow, J. B., Vaugh, H.: Central venous pressure monitoring. Rev Surg **24**, 163 (1967).

67. De Boscoli, G.: Veias subclavias e troncos venosas Dracquiocephalicos, novasvias de aceso para as transfusoes endovenosas. Pediatria (Rio de J), **21**, 113 (1956).

68. Bradley, M. N.: A technique for prolonged intraarterial catheterization. Surg Gynecol Obstet **119**, 117 (1964).

69. Brandt, R. K., Foley, W. J., Fink, G. H., Regan, W. J.: Mechanism of perforation of the heart

with production of hydropericardium by a venous catheter and its prevention. Am J Surg **119**, 311 (1970).

70. Brennan, M.F., Sugarbaker, P.H., Moore, F.P.: Venobronchial fistula a rare complication of central venous catheterization for parenteral nutrition. Arch Surg **106**, 871 (1973).

71. Brinkmann, A.J., Costley, D.O.: Internal jugular venepuncture. JAMA **223**, 182 (1973).

72. Briscoe, C.E., Buschmann, J.A., McDonald, W.J.: Extensive neurological damage after cannulation of internal jugular vein. Br Med J **1974/I** 314.

73. Brisman, R., Parks, L.C., Benson, D.W.: Pitfalls in the clinical use of central venous pressure. Arch Surg **95**, 902 (1967).

74. Brøckner, J.: Intravenous fluid therapy through a catheter inserted percutaneously in surgical patients. Acta Chir Scand **128**, 362 (1964).

75. Broviac, J.W., Cole, B.S., Schribner, B.H.: A silicone rubber atrial catheter for prolonged parenteral alimentation. Surg Gynecol Obstet **136**, 602 (1973).

76. Brown, C.A., Kent, A.: Perforation of right ventricle by polyethylene catheter. South Med J **49**, 466 (1956).

77. Brücke, P., Kucher, K., Steinbereithner, K., Wagner, O.: Technik und Ergebnisse des perkutanen V. Cava-inferior-Katheters bei 100 Patienten einer Intensivpflegestation. Z Prakt Anaesth **1**, 319 (1966).

78. Buchman, R.J.: Subclavian venepuncture. Milit Med **134**, 451 (1969).

79. Buchsmann, H.J., White, A.J.: The use of subclavian central catheters in gynecology and obstetrics. Surg Gynecol Obstet **136**, 561 (1973).

80. Burri, C., Müller, W.: Venendruckmessung im Tierversuch und beim chirurgischen Patienten. Anaesthesist **15**, 132 (1966).

81. Burri, C., Allgöwer, M.: Methodik der Venendruckmessung. Schweiz Med Wschr **96**, 624 (1966).

82. Burri, C., Kuner, E.: Bestimmung des zentralen Venendruckes in der Chirurgie. Med Neuheiten **72**, 81 (1966).

83. Burri, C., Allgöwer, M.: Klinische Erfahrungen mit der Messung des ZVD. Schweiz Med Wochenschr **97**, 1414 (1967).

84. Burri, C.: Kriterien zur Beurteilung hypovolämischer Zustände. Schweiz Z Militärmed **44**, 3 (1967).

85. Burri, C.: Der Vena cava-Katheter. Med Neuheiten **74**, 1 (1968).

86. Burri, C.: Der zentrale Venendruck. St. Gallen: Hausmann 1970.

87. Burri, C.: Die einfachen Kreislaufgrößen beim chirurgischen Patienten. Berlin-Heidelberg-New York: Springer 1971.

88. Burri, C., Gasser, D.: Der Vena-cava-Katheter. Berlin-Heidelberg-New York: Springer 1971.

89. Burri, C., Forberg, C.: Ein neues Kathetermodell zur parenteralen Ernährung. Infusionstherapie **2**, 63 (1973).

90. Burri, C.: Der Katheterismus der Vena cava. Wissenschaftliche Schriftreihe, Heft 8, St. Gallen: Hausmann 1975.

91. Burri, C., Krischak, G.: Fehler und Gefahren in der Anwendungstechnik der parenteralen Ernährung. Klin. Anaesth. u. Intensivtherapie Vol. 7, Berlin-Heidelberg-New York: Springer 1975.

92. Burri, C., Krischak, G.: Technik und Gefahren des Cava-Katheters. Infusionstherapie **3**, 174 (1976).

93. Busse, J., Schramm, G.: Intrathorakale Cavakatheterperforation. Prakt. Anaesth **9**, 48 (1974).

94. Carle, J.: Le problème des perfusions de longue durée. Concours Méd **89**, 6119 (1967).

95. Carney, Th.J.: Radiographic localization of central venous pressure catheter embolism. Report of a case. J Am Osteopath Assoc **71**, 351 (1971).

96. Chalmers, J.A., Fawns, H.T.: Prolonged anuria treated by infusion into the vena cava. Lancet **1955/I**, 79.

97. Chambers, J.W., Smith, G.: The use of caval catheterization in cases of severe oliguria and anuria. Brit J Surg **45**, 160 (1957).

98. Chase, St.P.: Hydrothorax complicating subclavian vein infusion therapy. Ohio State Med J **70**, 106 (1974).

99. Cheney, F.W., Lincoln, J.R.: Phlebitis from plastic intravenous catheters. Anaesthesiology **25**, 650 (1964).

100. Chodkiewicz, J.P., Creissard, P., Dehouve, P.: Migration intracardiaque d'un cathéter de perfusion intraveineuse découverte à l'autopsie d'un traumatisme cranien. Méd Lég domnage corpor **2**, 191 (1969).

101. Christensen, K.H., Nerstrom, B., Baden, H.: Complications of percutaneous catheterization of the subclavian vein in 129 cases. Acta Chir Scand **133**, 615 (1967).

102. Clauss, D.: Unsere Erfahrungen mit dem Subclavia-Katheter in der Langzeitinfusionstherapie. Zbl Chir **5**, 159 (1969).

103. Coblentz, D.R.: Radiographic detection of plastic catheter embolus. Calif Med **105**, 357 (1966).

104. Cohn, J.N., Luria, M.H.: Studies in clinical shock and hypotension. The value of bedside hemodynamic observation. JAMA **190**, 891 (1964).

105. Collin, J., Collin, Ch., Constable, F.L., Johnston, J.D.A.: Infusion thrombophlebitis and infection with various cannulas. Lancet **1976/II**, 150.

106. Collins, R. U., Braun, P. A., Zinner, St. H., Kass, E. H.: Risk of local and systemic infection with polyethylene intravenous catheters. N Engl J Med **279**, 340 (1968).

107. Collins, R. U., Braun, P. A., Zinner, St. H., Kass, E. H.: Risk of local and systemic infection with polyethylene intravenous catheters. JAMA **185**, 146 (1971).

108. McConnal, R., Fox, R. T.: Experience with per-cutaneous internal jugular-innominate vein catheterization. Can Med Assoc J **117**, 1 (1972).

109. Copeland, E. M., Mac Fadyen, B. V., Dudrick, S. J.: Prevention of microbial catheter contamination in patients receiving parenteral hyperalimentation. South Med J **67**, 303 (1974).

110. Corwin, J. H., Moseley, Th.: Subclavian vene-puncture and central venous pressure. Am Surg **32**, 413 (1966).

111. Craig, B.: Air embolus via CVP catheter without positive pressure. Ann Surg **179**, 479 (1974).

112. Craig, R. G., Jones, R. A., Sproul, G. J., Kinyon, G. E.: The alternate methods of central venous system catheterization Am Surg **34**, 131 (1968).

113. Cremer, W.: Herzperforation mit akuter Herztamponade bei Infusionskatheterisierung der Vena subclavia. Anaesth Prax **8**, 97 (1973).

114. Daily, P. O., Griepp, R. B., Shumway, N. E.: Percutaneous internal jugular vein cannulation. Arch Surg **101**, 534 (1969).

115. Dangel, P.: Die Technik der Infusionsbehandlung und der parenteralen Ernährung bei Neugeborenen und Säuglingen. Infusionstherapie **2**, 34 (1975).

116. Darvan, A.: The anatomy of intraclavicular subclavian vein-catheterization and its complications. Surg Gynecol Obstet **136**, 71 (1973).

117. Darrell, J. H., Garrod, L. P.: Secondary septicaemia from intravenous cannulae. Br Med J **1969/II**, 481.

118. Davidson, J. T., Ben Hur, N., Nathen, H.: Subclavian venepuncture. Lancet **1963/II**, 1139.

119. Defalque, R. J.: Subclavian venepuncture: A review. Anaesth Analg Curr Res **47**, 677 (1968).

120. Defalque, R. J.: The subclavian route. A critical review of the world literature up to 1970. Anaesthesist **21**, 325 (1972).

121. Defalque, R. J., Wittig, B.: Punktion und Katheterisierung der Vena jugularis interna. Anaesthesist **23**, 41 (1974).

122. Defalque, R. J.: Fatal complications of subclavian catheter. Can Anaesth Soc J **18**, 681 (1974).

123. Delany, D. J., Starer, F.: Recovery of catheters lost in vascular system. Br Med J **1972/I**, 510

124. Deubzner, W., Kia-Noury, M.: Praktische Bedeutung der Vena anonyma für Injektionen und Punktionen. Münch Med Wschr **107**, 1054 (1965).

125. Dhurandhar, R. W., Quiroz, A. C., De Pasquale, N. P., Burch, G. E.: The lack of influence of end and side orifices in cardiac catheters on venous pressure recording. Am Heart J **74**, 733 (1967).

126. Dickerson, M. E.: Hospital liable for loss of catheter. Curr Res Anaesth **47**, 222 (1968).

127. Dietz, H., Weyer, K. H.: Venographische Untersuchungen bei Patienten mit Vena-Cava-Katheter. Anaesthesiologie und Wiederbelebung Vol. 13, Infusionstherapie. Berlin-Heidelberg-New York: Springer 1966.

128. Dillon, J. D., Schaffner, W., Van Way, Ch. W., Meng, H. C.: Septicaemia and total parenteral nutrition. JAMA **223**, 1341 (1973).

129. Dimakakos, P. B., Radakowic, D., Balle, A.: Zur Frage der Subclaviapunktion und ihrer Komplikationen. Schweiz Med Wschr **102**, 14 (1972).

130. Doering, R. B., Stemmer, E. A., Conolly, J. E.: Complications of indwelling venous catheters. Am J Surg **114**, 259 (1967).

131. McDonough, J. J., William, A., Altemeier, M. D.: Subclavian venous thrombosis secondary to indwelling catheters. Surg Gynecol Obstet **133**, 397 (1971).

132. Doolas, A.: Planning alimentation of surgical patients. Surg Clin North Am **50**, 103 (1970).

133. Dotter, Ch. T., Rösch, J., Bilbao, M. K.: Transluminal extraction of catheter and guide fragments from the heart and great vessels: 29 collected cases. Am J Roentgenol Radium Ther Nucl Med. **111**, 467 (1971).

134. Druskin, M. S., Siegel, P. D.: Bacterial contamination of indwelling intravenous polyethylene catheters. JAMA **185**, 966 (1963).

135. Dudrick, St. J., Wilmore, D. W., Vars, H. M., Rhoads, J. E.: Long-term total parenteral nutrition with growth, development and positive nitrogen balance. Surgery **64**, 134 (1968).

136. Duffy, B. J.: The clinical use of polyethylene tubing for intravenous therapy. Ann Surg **130**, 929 (1949).

137. Duma, R. J., Warner, J. F., Dalton, H. P.: Septicaemia from intravenous infusions. N Engl J Med **5**, 257 (1971).

138. Eastridge, C. E., Clemmons, E. E., Hughes, F. A., Prather, J. R.: Use of CVP in the management of circulatory failure. Am J Surg **32**, 121 (1966).

139. Eastridge, C. E., Hughes, F. A.: Central venous pressure monitoring. A useful aid in the management of shock. Am J Surg **114**, 648 (1967).

140. Eckert, R. W., Grünhagen, H., Seifert, W.: Symptome bakterieller Besiedlung von venösen Kathetern. Zbl Chir **100**, 163 (1975).

141. Edelstein, J.: Atraumatic removal of a

polyethylene catheter from the superior vena cava. Chest **57**, 381 (1970).

142. Eerola, D., Eerola, M., Scharlin, M., Kankinen, L., Kaukinen, S.: Der Vena subclavia-Katheter. Erfahrungen bei der Einführung der Methode. Anaesthesist **19**, 437 (1970).

143. Edwards, W. H.: A hazard of embolus associated with indwelling intravenous catheters. Surgery **53**, 818 (1963).

144. Edwards, W. H.: Intracath-embolus. A rare complication of indwelling catheters used for intravenous therapy. South Med J **56**, 1354 (1963).

145. Eggert, A.: Erfahrungen mit dem Katheterismus der oberen Hohlvene über eine perkutane infraclaviculäre Punktion der V. anonyma oder der V. subclavia. Bruns Beitr Klin Chir **220**, 515 (1973).

146. Eisterer, H., Marsoner, F.: Eine seltene Komplikation bei Infusion in die Vena subclavia. Anaesthesist **12**, 395 (1966).

147. Eisterer, H., Kutscha-Lissberg, E.: Der "direkte" Cava-superior-Katheter. Wien Med Wschr **118**, 213 (1968).

148. Emmrich, P.: Die Anwendung des Cava-Katheters in der pädiatrischen Intensivpflege. Mschr Kinderheilk **119**, 218 (1971).

149. English, I. C. W., Frew, R. M., Pigott, J. F., Zaki, M.: Percutaneous catheterization of the internal jugular vein. Anaesthesia **24**, 521 (1969).

150. Eriksen, S.: Purcutaneous infraclavicular subclavian puncture. Nord Med **86**, 1302 (1971).

151. Fassolt, A., Braun, U., Schnaub, S.: Klinische Erfahrungen mit dem infraclaviculären Venenkatheterismus. Schweiz Med Wochenschr **98**, 461 (1968).

152. Fassolt, A., Braun, U., Graber, M.: Gefahren des Katheters der oberen Hohlvene mit besonderer Berücksichtigung des infraclaviculären Zuganges. Helv Chir Acta **37**, 18 (1970).

153. Fassolt, A., Schaefler, O., Braun, U.: Medikamentöse Maßnahmen gegen Begleitthrombosen bei Cavakathetern. Anaesthesist **22**, 324 (1973).

154. Fassolt, A. Neuere Aspekte der Sicherheit beim Vena-Cava-Katheter unter Berücksichtigung der Erfahrungen mit der Vena-Subclavia-Route. Schweiz Ass Zeitung **3**, 4 (1976).

155. Feiler, E. M., De Alva, W. E.: Infraclavicular percutaneous subclavian vein puncture. Am J Surg **118**, 996 (1969).

156. Felsch, G., Richter, G.: Subclaviakatheterismus. Z Ges Inn Med, Tagungsber **9**, 153 (1974).

157. Fenn, J. E., Stansel, H. C.: Certain hazards of the central venous catheter. Angiology **20**, 38 (1969).

158. Ferrer, J. M.: Fatal air embolism via subclavian vein. N Engl J Med **282**, 688 (1970).

159. Ffaracs, J. H.: Central venous thrombosis following central venous catheterization and parenteral nutrition. NZ Med J **81**, 420 (1975).

160. Fidgor, P. P.: Die Technik des Cava-Katheters. Wien Klin Wochenschr **73**, 69 (1961).

161. Filler, R. M., Eraklis, A. J., Rubin, V. G.: Longterm parenteral nutrition in infants. N Engl J Med **281**, 589 (1969).

162. Finley, R. K.: Vena cava infusion. Med Times **89**, 373 (1961).

163. Firor, H. V.: Pulmonary embolization complicating total intravenous alimentation. J Pediatr. Surg **7**, 81 (1972).

164. Fischer, F., Dietz, H., Halmágyi, M.: Klinische Erfahrungen mit dem Vena-Cava-Katheter. Anaesthesiologie und Wiederbelebung Vol. 13 Infusionstherapie.   Berlin-Heidelberg-New York: Springer, 1966.

165. Fisher, R. G., Romero, J. R.: Extraction of an embolized venous catheter using percutaneous technique. Radiology **116**, 735 (1975).

166. Fitts, Ch. T., Barnett, L. Th., Webb, C. M., Sexton, J., Yarbrough, D. R.: Perforating wounds of the heart caused by central venous catheters. J Trauma **10**, 764 (1970).

167. Flanagan, J. P., Gradisar, J. A.: Air embolism. Complication of subclavian venepuncture. N Engl J Med **281**, 488 (1969).

168. Flanagan, J. P., Gradisar, J. A., Gross, R. I., Kelly, Th. R.: Air embolus — a lethal complication of subclavian venepuncture. N Engl J Med **281**, 489 (1969).

169. Forssmann, W.: Die Sondierung des rechten Herzens, Klin Wschr **8**, 2085 (1929).

170. Fontanelle. L. J., Dooley, B. N., Cuello, L.: Subclavian venepuncture and its complications. Ann Thorac Surg **11**, 331 (1971).

171. Franke, H., Opderbecke, H. W.: Die Bedeutung einer Wachstation in der Überwachung und Behandlung Frischoperierter. Chirurg **30**, 487 (1959).

172. Freeman, R., King, B.: Infective complications of indwelling intravenous catheters and the monitoring of infections by the nitrobluetetrazolium-Test. Lancet **1972 I**, 992.

173. Freeman, J. B., Davis, P. L., MacLean, L. D.: Candida endophthalmitis associated with intravenous hyperalimentation. Arch Surg **108**, 237 (1974).

174. Friedländer, K.: Erfahrungen mit dem Subclavia-Katheter in einem mittleren Krankenhaus. Dtsch Med Wochenschr **97**, 1602 (1972).

175. Friedmann, E. F., Grable, E., Fine, J.: Central venous pressure and direct serial measurements as guides in blood volume replacement. Lancet **1966 II**, 609.

176. Friedmann, B. A., Jurguleit, H. C.: Perforation of atrium by polyethylene CV-Catheter. JAMA **203**, 1141 (1968).

Royer, P., Pellerin, D.: Alimentation parentérale continuée par cahtéter intracave chez
l'enfant. Ann Chir Infant Parm **13**, 7 (1972).

396. Rolle, J.: Vergleichende Untersuchungen zur
Oberflächenbeurteilung von Kunststoffverweilkanülen. Bruns Beitr Klin Chir **219**, 468
(1972).

397. Ronk, R.: Weichmacher im Blut. Eur Med **3**,
22 (1971).

398. Ross, A. M.: Polyethylene emboli: How many
more? Chest **57**, 307 (1970).

399. Ross, J. K.: Vena caval infusion. Postgrad Med
J **33**, 623 (1957).

400. Ross, S. A.: Infusion phlebitis; selected factors.
Nurs Res **21**, 313 (1972).

401. Rossi, P.: "Hook catheter" technique for transfemoral removal of foreign body from the right
side of the heart. Am J Roentgenol Radium
Ther Nucl. Med **109**, 101 (1970).

402. Royal, H. O., Shieldes, J. B., Donati, R. M.:
Misplacement of central venous pressure catheters and unilateral pulmonary edema. Arch Intern Med **135**, 1502 (1975).

403. Ryan, G. M., Howland, W. S.: An evaluation of
central venous pressure monitoring. Anaesth
Analg Curr Res **45**, 754 (1966).

404. Ryan, J. A.: Catheter complications in total
parenteral nutrition. N Engl J Med **290**, 757
(1974).

405. Sabuncu, N., Volles, E., Gressner, P., Prill, A.,
Harms, U.: Pathologisch-anatomische Befunde
und haemodynamische Grundlagen bei Anwendung des Vena subclavia-Katheters. Dtsch
Z Nervenheilkd **196**, 266 (1969).

406. Saegesser, M.: Die Bedeutung des zentralen
venösen Blutdruckes in der Chirurgie. Schweiz
Med Wochenschr **95**, 974 (1965).

407. Salo, E. L., Eerola, R., Eerola, M.: Der Vena-
Subclavia-Katheter bei Kindern. Z Kinderchir
12, 3 (1973).

408. Scebat, L., Renais, J., Meeus-Bith, L., Le
Nègre, J.: Accidents, indications et contreindication du cathéterisme des cavités droites du
cœur. Arch Mal Cœur **50**, 943 (1957).

409. Schaeffer, H.: Eine neue Methode zur Bestimmung des zentralen Venendruckes beim
Menschen. Klin Wochenschr **31**, 802 (1953).

410. Schaeffer, H.: Zur Frage der Vena anonyma-
Punktion als Zugangsweg für Infusionen und
Transfusionen. Anaesthesist **16**, 303 (1968).

411. Schapira, M., Sterin, W. Z.: Hazards of subclavian vein cannulation for central venous
pressure monitoring. JAMA **201**, 111 (1967).

412. Scharf, F. L., Berman, B. J., Cleveland, E. D.:
Some complications in the use of indwelling in-
travenous polyethylene catheters. Med. Serv.
J. Can. **15**, 724 (1959).

413. Schechter, E., Parisi, A. F.: Removal of catheter fragments from pulmonary artery using
a snare. Br Heart J **34**, 699 (1972).

414. Schlag, G.: Die Bedeutung des zentralen Venendruckes in der Traumatologie. Chirurg **38**,
523 (1967).

415. Schlarb, K.: Subclaviapunktion. Anaesthesist
21, 477 (1972).

416. Schloßmann, D.: Thrombogenic properties of
vascular catheter materials in vivo. Radiology
91, 251 (1968).

417. Schmidt, Ch., Teucher, H. J.: Die Katheterisierung der Vena subclavia als Bestandteil
der Intensivtherapie. Z Aerztl Fortbild **65**, 367
(1971).

418. Schmitz, E. R., Martin, E., Keller, P.: Grundlagen der Venenpunktion. Infusionstherapie **3**,
180 (1976).

419. Schöche, J.: Der Subclavia-Katheter in der
chirurgischen Intensivtherapie. Zbl Chir **98**,
270 (1973).

420. Scholz, G., Loewe, K. R.: Die Punktion der
Vena subclavia und ihre Komplikationen aus
pathologischanatomischer Sicht. Med Welt **20**,
2248 (1969).

421. Schulte, H. D.: Anatomische und technische
Möglichkeiten der intravenösen Infusionsbehandlung. Dtsch. Med. Wochenschr. **94**,
1793 (1969).

422. Schumann, G.: Die Komplikationen bei der
Anwendung sog. zentraler Venenkatheter aus
pathologisch-anatomischer Sicht. Z Kreislaufforsch **60**, 355 (1971).

423. Schweikert, C. H., Grünagel, H. H.: Doppelseitiger Pleuraerguß bei Infusionstherapie
am Hals. Thoraxchirurgie **11**, 421 (1964).

424. Shander, D.: Removal of an embolized
polyethylene catheter using an uretral stone
catheter. Chest **57**, 318 (1970).

425. Shang, N. G. W., Rosen, M.: Positioning central
venous catheters through the basilic vein.
A comparison of catheters. Br J Anaesth **45**,
1211 (1973).

426. Shenkin, H. A.: On the diagnosis of hemorrhage in man. Am J Sci **4**, 421 (1944).

427. Siewert, R., Bauers, S., Wiek, K., Bortfeldt, K.:
Bakterielle Komplikationen beim Venenkatheterismus. Dtsch Med J **21**, 333 (1970).

428. Silberschmid, M., Saito, S., Smitz, L. L.: Circulatory effects of acute latic acidosis in dogs
prior and after hemorrhage. J Surg. **112**, 175
(1966).

429. Simon, J.: Praxis und Technik der parenteralen
Ernährung. Prakt Anaesth **11**, 146 (1976).

430. Smith, B. E., Modell, H. J., Gaub, M. L., Moya,
F.: Complications of subclavian vein catheterization. Arch Surg **90**, 228 (1965).

431. Smithwick, W., Stalheim, G. K., Love, J. W.:
Removal of foreign bodies from the superior
vena cava and right atrium without
thoracotomy. Ann Thorac Surg **17**, 197 (1974).

432. Smits, H., Freedman, L. R.: Prolonged venous

Punktion der Vena jugularis interna, ein neuer Zugangsweg zur Vena cava superior. Anaesth Inform **2**, 67 (1963).

216. Heitmann, D.: Dosierungs- und Anwendungsrichtlinien für die intravenöse Zufuhr von Nährstoffen im Rahmen der Langzeiternährung bei Nichttraumatisierten. Klin. Anaesth. u. Intensivtherapie Vol. 7. Berlin-Heidelberg-New York: Springer 1975.

217. Heitmann, D., Regler, G.: Die Vena jugularis interna als Zugangsweg für den Cava-Katheter. Klinikarzt **5**, 331 (1976).

218. Helmer, F.: Iatrogene Fremdkörper in Herz und Lungen. Thoraxchirurgie **44**, 664 (1969).

219. Helmer, F., Vécsei, V.: Iatrogener Fremdkörper im rechten Herzen infolge Spiralabrisses beim Anlegen eines oberen Hohlvenenkatheters im Rahmen der Intensivpflege. Z. Prakt Anaesth **8**, 173 (1973).

220. Hemmer, R.: Complications relating to ventricularvenous shunts: A five year study. Dev Med Child Neurol **15**, 228 (1968).

221. Hemswald, R. R., Bwins, B. A., Griffen, W. O.: Analysis of safety factors in percutaneous deep venous cannulation. JAMA **127**, 623 (1974).

222. Henley, F. T., Ballard, J. W.: Percutaneous removal of lexible foreign body from the heart. Radiology **92**, 176 (1969).

223. Henneberg, U., Schröder, M.: Zur Problematik der Vena cava-Katheter. Chirurg **36**, 180 (1965).

224. Henneberg, U., Schröder, M.: Komplikationen beim Vena cava-Katheter. Anaesthesiologie und Wiederbelebung, Vol. 13, Infusionstherapie. Berlin-Heidelberg-New York: Springer 1966.

225. McHenry, M. M., Hopkins, D. M.: Cardiac tamponade as a result of infusion. JAMA **203**, 167 (1968).

226. Hentschel, M.: Vena cava-Katheter via Vena jugularis externa bei schweren chirurgischen Erkrankungen zur i. v. Substitution und Blutdiagnostik. Langenbecks Arch Chir **308**, 486 (1964).

227. Henzel, J. H., De Weege, U. S.: Morbid and mortal complications associated with prolonged central venous cannulation. Am J Surg **121**, 600 (1971).

228. Herbert, W. H., Sobol, B. J., Rohmann, M., Lubetsky, H. W., Rodriquez, V., Morsh, J. H. C.: Angiographic visualization of polyethylene catheter embolus. NY State J Med **69**, 316 (1969).

229. Hermoshura, B., Vanags, L., Dickey, M. W.: Measurement of pressure during intravenous therapy. JAMA **195**, 321 (1966).

230. Heunisch, K., Engelmann, L., Wildführ, W., Kühler, H.: Erfahrungen mit intravenösen Verweilkathetern bei internen Erkrankungen. Dtsch Gesundheitsw **27**, 1462 (1972).

231. Hildebrandt, J.: Zur perkutanen Katheterisation der Vena cava-superior von der Ellenbeuge aus. Z Ärztl. Fortbild **67**, 1199 (1973).

232. Hildebrandt, J., Schaps, P., Mikulin, H. D.: Ein tierexperimenteller Vergleich von unpräparierten, siliconisierten und "heparingequollenen" PVC-Schläuchen. Z Exp Chir **7**, 94 (1974).

233. Hildebrandt, J., Mukulin, H. D.: Thromboserisiko bei antithrombogenen Venenkathetern. Zbl Chir **100**, 159 (1975).

234. Hill, G. J.: Central venous pressure technique. Surg Clin North Am. **49**, 1351 (1969).

235. Hiotakis, K., Kronberger-Schönecker: Indikationen, Vorteile und Komplikationen des Vena cava-Katheters unter besonderer Berücksichtigung der Punktion des Angulus venosus. Zbl Chir **98**, 263 (1973).

236. Hipona, F. A., Sciammas, F. D., Hublitz, U. F.: Nonthoracotomy retrieval of intraluminal cardiovascular foreign bodies. Radiol Chlin North Am **9**, 583 (1971).

237. Hodel, H. L.: Transfemoral rescue of lost intravascular catheters and guide wires. J Can Assoc Radiol **24**, 42 (1973).

238. Hohn, A. R., Lamert, E. C.: Continous venous catheterization in children. JAMA **197**, 140 (1966).

239. Holder, T. M., Crow, M. L.: Free intracardiac foreign body; complication of ventriculo-atrial shunt for hydrocephalus. J Thorac Cardiovasc Surg **45**, 138 (1963).

240. Holt, H. M.: Central venous pressure via peripheral veins. Anaesthesiology **28**, 1093 (1967).

241. Homesley, H. D., Zelenik, J. S.: Hazards of central venous pressure monitoring; pericardial tamponade. Surg Gynecol Obstet **130**, 520 (1970).

242. Horisberger, B.: Die Bedeutung der kontinuierlichen Überwachung des zentralen Venendruckes bei labilen Kreislaufverhältnissen. Helv Chir Acta **33**, 9 (1966).

243. Horisberger, B.: Infektiöse Komplikationen durch Venenkatheter und deren Prophylaxe. Helv Chir Acta **34**, 21 (1967).

244. Hoskins, P. A., Mich, A. A., Ause, R. G.: Fibrin sleeve formation on indwelling subclavian central venous catheters. Arch Surg **102**, 353 (1971).

245. Hoshal, V. L.: Total intravenous nutrition with peripherally inserted silicone elastomer central venous catheters. Arch Surg **110**, 644 (1975).

246. Hossli, G.: Die praktische Bedeutung der Venendruckmessung bei Notfällen. Z Unfallmed Berufskr **2**, 97 (1965).

247. Hossli, G., Burri, C.: Manometrie im Schock. Klin Med **22**, 21 (1967).

248. Hughes, R. E., Magovern, G. J.: The relationship between right atrial pressure and blood-volume. Arch Surg **79**, 239 (1959).

249. Huth, J.H., Kalkowski, H., Schultz, J., Schwarz, F.: Zur Therapie der Katheterembolien. Zbl Chir **98**, 1365 (1973).
250. Hyman, A.L.: An improved snare catheter for retrieving fragments of polyethylene tubing. Chest **62**, 98 (1972).
251. Indar, R.: The danger of indwelling polyethylene cannulae in deep veins. Lancet I, **1959 I**, 284.
252. Irmer, W.: Entfernung eines embolisch von der linken Cubitalvene eingeschwemmten Polyaethylenkatheters aus dem Pulmonalisstamm. Zbl Chir **89**, 1078 (1964).
253. Ithot, Z., Carlton, N., Lucien, H.W., Shally, A.V.: Long term plastic tube implantation into the external jugular vein for injection or infusion in the dog. Surgery **66**, 768 (1969).
254. Jaeger, G.H., Cowly, R.A.: Studies on the use of polythene as a fibrous tissue stimulant. Ann Surg **128**, 509 (1948).
255. Jaeger, R.J., Rubin, R.J.: Plasticizers from plastic devices: Extraction, metabilism and accumulation by biological systems. Science **170**, 460 (1970).
256. Jaikaran, S.M.: Normal central venous pressure. Br J Srg **55**, 609 (1968).
257. James, P.M.: Clinical uses of central venous cannulation. Postgrad Med **55**, 155 (1974).
258. Jenkins, I.C., Screech, G.: Central venous pressure monitoring in anaesthesia. Can Anaesth Soc J **13**, 513 (1966).
259. Jernigan, W.R., Gardner, W.C., Mahr, M.N., Milburn, J.L.: Use of the internal jugular vein for placement of central venous catheter. Surg Gynecol Obstet **130**, 520 (1970).
260. Jernigan, W.R., Gardner, W.C., Mahr, M.N., Milburn, J.L.: The internal jugular vein for access to the central venous system. JAMA **218**, 97 (1971).
261. Johnson, Ch.C., Lazarchick, J., Lynn, M.B.: Subclavian venepunctures: Preventable complications, report of two cases. Mayo Clin Proc **45**, 712 (1970).
262. Johnson, Ch.C.: Perforation of right atrium by a polyethylene catheter. JAMA **195**, 854 (1966).
263. Johnson, L.M., Gillis, S.P., Lynn, H.B.: Unusual complication of intravenous fluid therapy. Surgery **53**, 809 (1963).
264. Jones, M.V., Craig, D.B.: Venous reaction to plastic intravenous cannulae. Can Anaesth Soc J **19**, 491 (1972).
265. Jones, R.R.: Venous pressure in general anaesthesia. Anaesth Analg Curr Res **42**, 470 (1963).
266. Käufer, C., Savice, B.: Risiken venöser Dauerkatheter. Langenbecks Arch Chir **65**, 1022 (1972).
267. Kahl, Ch.: Punktion und Sondierung der Vena subclavia. Anaesth Prax **8**, 79 (1973).
268. Kahl, Ch.: Punktion und Sondierung der Vena subclavia. Internist Prax **14**, 85 (1974).
269. Keddie, N.C., Provan, J.L., Austen, W.G.: Central venous pressure, blood volume determinations and the effect of vasoactive drugs in hypovolemic shock. Surgery **60**, 427 (1966).
270. Keenleyside, H.B.: External jugular vein for rapid transfusion during surgery. Can Anaesth Soc J **9**, 512 (1962).
271. Keeri-Szanto, M.: The subclavian vein, a constant intravenous injection site. Arch Surg **72**, 179 (1956).
272. Keeri-Szanto, M.: La voie veineuse sousclaviculaire en anaesthesie. Can Anaesth Soc J **4**, 55 (1957).
273. Keßler, E.: Die Katheterembolie. Zbl Chir **98**, 989 (1973).
274. Khalil, K.G., Parker, F.B., Mukherjee, N., Webb, W.R.: Thoracic duct injury. A complication of jugular vein catheterization. JAMA **221**, 908 (1972).
275. Kleinschmidt, E., Marx, E.: Oberer Cava-Katheter via vena cephalica dextra sive sinistra. Med Welt **23**, 719 (1972).
276. Kline, J.K., Hofman, W.J.: Cardiac tamponade from CVP-catheter perforation. JAMA **206**, 1794 (1968).
277. Klötzer, B., Mlynek, H.J.: Die Cava-Katheterembolie – eine seltene Komplikation bei der Anwendung von Cava-Kathetern. Zbl Chir **94**, 1085 (1969).
278. Kluge, W.: Beitrag zur peripheren Katheterembolie. Z Ärztl Fortbild **68**, 895 (1974).
279. Knutson, H., Sternberg, K.: Pulmonary embolus with foreign body in case of fractured femoral catheter. Nord Med **62**, 1491 (1959).
280. Knutson, H., Sternberg, K.: Lungemboli due to breatzing of catheter (in Swedish) Nord Med **62**, 1491, 1959).
281. Koch, M.J.: Bilateral i. v. hydrothorax. N Engl J Med **286**, 218 (1972).
282. Kösters, B., Bartels, D.: Erfahrungen mit der Subclaviakatheterisierung auf der Wachstation. Med Ernähr **11**, 63 (1970).
283. Konold, R., Ullmann, U., Schrader, C.P., Kieninger, G.: Klinische und bakteriologische Beobachtungen bei intravenös eingeführten Kathetern. Dtsch Med Wochenschr **99**, 1009 (1974).
284. Krischak, G., Burri, C.: Klinische und physikalische Untersuchungen über die Abhängigkeit der Komplikationen vom Material des Cava-Katheters. Langenbecks Arch Chir Forum 1974, 167.
285. Kröpelin, K., Mössner, G., Gebhardt, W.: Lubclaviakatheter als Streuherd bei Pilzsepsis. Dtsch Med Wochenschr **93**, 1098 (1968).
286. Kucher, R., Steinbereithner, K.: Intensivstation, Intensivpflge, Intensivtherapie. Stuttgart: Thieme 1972.

287. Kuhn, W., Bach, H.G.: Punktion und Katheterismus der Vena subclavia in Geburtshilfe und Gynäkologie. Geburtshilfe Frauenheilkd. **26**, 1272 (1966).
288. Kuiper, D.H.: Cardiac tamponade and death in a patient receiving total parenteral nutrition. JAMA **230**, 877 (1974).
289. Kurock, W., Schier, J.: Erfahrungen mit dem Vena cava-Katheter. Med Welt **25**, 135 (1974).
290. Kux, M., Kutscha-Lissberg, E.: Die Gefahr der Katheterembolie beim oberen Hohlvencn-kathcter. Anaesthesist **17**, 232 (1968).
291. Ladd, M., Schreiner, G.E.: Plastic tubing for intravenous alimentation. JAMA **145**, 642 (1951).
292. Lamprecht, W.: Clinical aspects of iatrogenic intra cardiac foreign bodies. Chirurg **36**, 182 (1965).
293. Lamprecht, W.: Zur Kasuistik iatrogener intrakardialer Fremdkörper. Chirurg **36**, 182 (1965).
294. Land, R.E.: Anatomic relationship of the right subclavian vein. Arch. Surg **102**, 178 (1971).
295. Land, R.E.: The relationship of the left subclavian vein to the clavicle. J Thorac Cardiovasc Surg **63**, 564 (1972).
296. Landis, E.M., Hortenstine, J.C.: Functional significance of venous blood pressure. Physiol Rev **30**, 1 (1950).
297. Lang, H.: Venae sectio und Cava-Katheter. a) Anästh Prax **2**, 141 (1967). b) Pädiatr Prax **7**, 443 (1968). c) Intern Prax **8**, 297 (1968).
298. Lanz, T., Wachsmut, W.: Praktische Anatomie. Berlin-Heidelberg-New York: Springer 1955.
299. Larsen, H.W., Lindahl, F.: Lesion of the internal mamarian artery caused by infraclavicular percutaneous catheterization of the subclavian vein. Acta Chir Scand **139**, 571 (1973).
300. Lassner, J.: Französiche Erfahrungen mit der parenteralen Ernährung. Parenterale Ernährung. Lang, Frey, Halmágyi (eds.): Berlin-Heidelberg-New York: Springer, 1966.
301. Lavigne, J.E., Brown, C.S., Machiedo, G.W.: Improved technique for long-term venous catheterization. J Am Surg **127**, 624 (1974).
302. Lawin, P.: Praxis der Intensivbehandlung. Stuttgart: Thieme 1968.
303. McLean, L.D.: Blood volume versus central venous pressure in shock. Surg Gynecol Obstet **118**, 594 (1964).
304. McLean, L.D.: Treatment of shock in man based on hemodynamic diagnosis. Surg Gynecol Obstet **120**, 1 (1965).
305. Leiss, F., Peter, K.H.: Die Silicone in Medizin, Pharmazie und Lebensmittelindustrie. Arzneimittelforschung **4**, 571 (1954).
306. Lemon, V.: Cannulation of the inferior vena cava as the last posibility of a venous approach. Rozhl Chir **53**, 745 (1974).
307. Leth, A., Ehlers, D., Jensen, G., Lauridsen, P.: Removal of a catheter fragment from the right atrium by a new catheterization technique. Scand J Thorac Cardiovasc Surg **7**, 171 (1973).
308. Levinsky, W.J.: Fatal air embolis during insertion of CVP monitoring apparatus. JAMA **209**, 1721 (1969).
309. Levy, N.M.: The cardiovascular physiology of the critically ill patient. Surg Clin North Am **55**, 483 (1975).
310. Lillehei, C.W., Bonnabeau, R.C., Grossling, S.: Removal of iatrogenic foreign bodies within cardiac chambers and great vessels. Circulation **32**, 782 (1965).
311. Lindenberg, I., Gjorup, S., Aagaard, P.: Parenteral fluid administration through a catheter inserted into the inferior vena cava. Acta Chir Scand **117**, 342 (1959).
312. Linder, M.M.: Vena subclavia-Katheterisierung. Fortschr Med **91**, 659 (1973).
313. Loers, F.J., Pesendorfer, H.: Perforation einer Pulmonalarterie – eine seltene Komplikation der Cava-Katheter. Z Prakt Anaesth **8**, 315 (1973).
314. Loers, F.J.: Der obere Hohlvenenkatheter über die Vena jugularis interna. Chirurg **45**, 333 (1974).
315. Loers, F.J.: Probleme des intravenösen Zugangs – ein neues Besteck für den Cava-Katheter über die Vena jugularis interna. Infusionstherapie **3**, 34 (1976).
316. Loers, F.J., Lindau, B., Walter, E.: Extraktion eines abgeschnittenen Cava-Katheters mit einem Steinfänger. Chirurg **47**, 246 (1976).
317. Lohmöller, G., Bauer, H., Ruhwinkel, B., Kaiser, W., Lydtin, H.: Herzbeuteltamponade während parentreraler Ernährung über einen Subclavia-Katheter. Münch Med Wochenschr **117**, 1463 (1975).
318. Longerbeam, J.K., Vannix, R., Wagner, W.: Central venous pressure monitoring. Am J Surg **110**, 220 (1965).
319. Lowenbraun, St., Young, V., Kenton, D., Serpick, A.A.: Infection from intravenous "scalp-vein" needles in a susceptible population. JAMA **212**, 451 (1970).
320. Lucas, Ch.E.: Air embolus via subclavian catheter. N Engl J Med **281**, 966 (1968).
321. Lutz, H.: Pathophysiologie der zentralen Venendruckmessung. In: Anaesthesiologie und Wiederbelebung Vol. 34, Venendruckmessung. Berlin-Heidelberg-New York: Springer 1968.
322. Lutz, H.: Differenzierung verschiedener Formen des Schocks durch einfache Meßverfahren. Dtsch Med Wochensch **91**, 1043 (1966).
323. Mahaffey, J.E., Witherspoon, S.M.: An unusual complication following venous cutdown. Anesthesiologie **27**, 198 (1966).
324. Malinak, L.R., Gulde, R.E., Faris, A.M.: Percutaneous subclavian catheterization for central

venous pressure monitoring. Am J Obstet Gynecol **92**, 477 (1965).

325. Makarov, V. S., Osipov, A. P., Lybin, I. U. M.: Percutaneous puncture catheterization of the subclavian vein. Klin Khir **11**, 65 (1974).

326. Mariano, B. P., Roper, C. L., Staple, T. W.: Accidental migration of an intravenous catheter from the arm to the lung. Radiology **86**, 736 (1966).

327. Markkula, H., Baer, G., Heldt, C., Isotalo, J., Väyrynen, J.: Entfernung eines abgeschnittenen Vena-subclavia-Katheters aus dem rechten Herzen mit Hilfe einer urologischen Faßzange. Anaesthesist **23**, 232 (1974).

328. Marlon, A. M., Cohn, L. H., Fogarty, Th. J., Harrison, D. C.: Retrieval of catheter fragments. Calif Med **115**, 61 (1971).

329. Massumi, R. A., Ross, A. M.: Atraumatic nonsurgical technique for removal of broken catheters from cardias cavities. N Engl J Med **277**, 195 (1967).

330. Mathey, J., Binet, J. P.: 7 cas de corps étrangers intrapéricardiques, intramyocardiques ou intracardiaques opérés. Presse Méd. **70**, 57 (1962).

331. Mathias, K.: Fehllagen von Venenkathetern. Dtsch Med Wochenschr **101**, 612 (1976).

332. Mathur, A. P., Pochaczersky, R., Levowith, B. S., Ferarn, F.: Fogarty balloon catheter for removal of catheter fragment in subclavian vein. JAMA **217**, 481 (1971).

333. Matz, R.: Complications of determining the central venous pressure. N Engl J Med **272**, 703 (1965).

334. Mauthe, H.: Removal of catheter embolus from right pulmonary artery. Wis Med J **72**, 151 (1973).

335. Meiel, G., Spithaler, W.: Vorzüge und Probleme des infraclavicularen Cavakatheters. Aktuel Probl Chir **10**, 149 (1975).

336. Meisner, H., Duswald, H.: Zur Infusionstechnik in der Intensivtherapie — Erfahrungen mit der Subclaviapunktion. Münch Med Wschr **114**, 861 (1972).

337. Meisner, H., Duswald, H.: Infusionstechnik im Schock. Anaesth Prax **8**, 137 (1973).

338. Melnick, St., Smith, D. E.: Candida tropicalis and torulopsis glabrata fungemia in a patient treated with long-term hyperalimentation. Am Surg. **40**, 190 (1974).

339. Merkel, F. K., McQuarrie, D. G.: Cutdown of the subclavian vein. Surgery **65**, 866 (1969).

340. Meyers, L.: Intravenous catheterization. Am J Nurs **45**, 930 (1945).

341. Miller, R. E., Cockerill, E. M., Isch, J. H.: Removal of intravascular and endobronchial foreign bodies by nonoperative snare technique. Surgery **69**, 463 (1971).

342. Mirhoseini, M., O'Connor, Th. M., Weisel, W.: Embolic catheter removed from pulmonary artery. JAMA **202**, 167 (1967).

343. Moncrief, J. A.: Femoral catheters. Ann Surg **147**, 166 (1958).

344. Moran, J. M., Altwood, R. P., Rowe, M. J.: A clinical and bacteriologic study of infections associated with venous cutdowns. N Engl J Med **272**, 554 (1965).

345. Morgan, M. G., Glasser, St. P.: Fixation of i. v. Catheters. N Engl J Med **291**, 1309 (1974).

346. Mühe, H., Bürger, L., Schellerer, W.: Venenkatheterembolie. Therapiewoche **20**, 2208 (1970).

347. Müller, C., Koch, P., Schahriari, Sch.: Bakteriologische Nachuntersuchungen bei Cava-Kathetern. Z Prakt Anaesth. **7**, 55 (1972).

348. Müller, K. M., Blaser, B.: Tödliche thromboembolische Komplikationen nach zentralem Venenkatheter. Dtsch Med Wschr **101**, 411 (1976).

349. Nachnani, G. H., Lessin, L. S., Motomiya, T., Jensen, W. N.: Scanning electron microscopy of thrombogenesis on vascular catheter surfaces. N Engl J Med **286**, 139 (1972).

350. Nager, F., Steinbrunn, W.: Therapie des kardiogenen Schocks nach Herzinfarkt. Schweiz Med Wochenschr. **97**, 389 (1967).

351. McNair, T. J., Dudley, H. A.: The local complications of intravenous therapy. Lancet **959/II**, 365.

352. Nasilowski, W., Meissner, A. J., Bukowska, O.: Dangers of long-term intravenous infusions with indwelling polyethylene catheters. Pol Tyg Lek **38**, 1470 (1973).

353. Nash, G., Moylan, J. S.: Paradoxical catheter embolism. Arch Surg **102**, 213 (1971).

354. Neegaard, J., Nielsen, B., Faburby, V.: Plasticizers in PVC and the occurrence of hepatitis in a hemodialysis unit. Scand J Urol Nephrol **5**, 141 (1971).

355. Niesel, H. C., Lee, P. F. S.: Punktion der Vena subclavia unter Verwendung von Teflonkathetern. Z. Prakt. Anaesth Wiederbeleb **7**, 170 (1972).

356. Nissen-Druey, C.: Iatrogene Fremdkörper-Embolie. Münch Med Wochenschr. **108**, 788 (1966).

357. Norden, C. W.: Application of antibiotic ointment to the site of venous catheterization — a controlled trial. J. Infect. Dis **120**, 611 (1969).

358. Nordlund, S., Thorén, L.: Catheter in the superior vena cava. Acta Chir **Scand 127**, 39 (1964).

359. Northcutt, C. E.: Intravenous loss of polyethylene catheters. Gen. Practitioner **34**, 125 (1966).

360. Nugent, R. P.: Supraclavicular catheterization of the subclavian vein. Aust NZ J Surg **43**, 41 (1973).

361. Obel,   I.W.P.:   Transient   phrenic-nerve paralysis following subclavian venepuncture. Anaesthesiology 33, 369, 1970.

362. Odmann, P.: The radiopaque polyethylene catheter. Acta Radiol (Stockh) 52, 64 (1959).

363. Oeri, H.U., Marty, H.: Langzeitkanülierung der Vena subclavia im Dienste der chirurgischen Intensivpflege. Helv Chir Acta 3, 221 (1971).

364. Opderbecke. H.W., Bardachzi, E.: Die Verwendung eines Cava-Katheters bei langdauernder Infusionsbehandlung. Dtsch Med Wochenschr. 86, 203 (1961).

365. Opderbecke, H.W., Bardachzi, E.: Erfahrungen mit der Anwendung eines Vena Cava-Katheters zur langfristigen Infusionstherapie bei 800 Kranken. Anaesthesiologie und Wiederbelebung Bd. 13, Infusionstherapie 1, 168, 1966.

366. Opderbecke, H.W., Bardachzi, E.: Problematik und Erfahrung bei der Anwendung eines Cava-Katheters zu Infusionszwecken. Z. Prakt. Anaesth Wiederbeleb 1, 239 (1966).

367. Opderbecke, H.W.: Indikation für die Wahl des Zugangsweges. Med Mitt 48, 173 (1974).

368. Orestano, F., Dietz, H.: Endophlebitis und Myocarditis als seltene Komplikation bei Anwendung von Vena-Cava-Kathetern. Anaesthesist 15, 225 (1966).

369. Otteni, J.C., Grandhaye, N., Dupeyron, J.P., Gauthier-Lafaye, J.P.: Deux complications fréquentes des cathéters veineux: Les fausses routes et les perforations vasculaires. Intérêt d'un controle radiographique systématique du cathéter. Anesth Analg (Paris) 28, 1149 (1971).

370. Pawlow, J.N., Gelfand, G.J., Ezlawa, N.W.: Transcutaneous catheterization of the subclavian vein. Chirurgie 12, 63 (1974).

371. Petty, W.C.: A simple technique for inserting catheters intravenously in difficult anatomic areas. Anesthesiology 39, 555, 1973.

372. Pierson, M., Lascombes, G., Pernot, C., Jeannin, B.: Asystolie irréductible due à la présence d'un cathéter en polythène dans les cavités cardiaques. Arch Fr Pédiatr 19, 231 (1962).

373. Polgerstorfer, H.W., Finkenstedt, G., Kleinberger, G., Kotzaurek, R.: Subclaviakatheter im Rahmen der internen Intensivmedizin. Wien Klin Wochenschr 50, 822, (1973).

374. Pässler, H.H., Burri, C.: Cavakatheterembolien. Helv Chir Acta 39, 613 (1972).

375. Pässler, H.H., Pfarr, B.: Komplikationen beim Cava-Katheterismus. Wehrmed Mschr 5, 140 (1973)

376. Parikh, R.K.: Horner's syndrome. A complication of percutaneous catheterization of internal jugular vein. Anaesthesia 27, 327 (1972).

377. Paskin, D.L., Hoffmann, W.S., Tuddenham, W.J.: A new complication ofsubclavian vein catheterization. Ann Surg 179, 266 (1974).

378. Paulet-Painboeuf, C.: 250 cathéterismes parcutanés de la veine jugulaire interne. Presse Méd 1, 1098 (1972).

379. Pokieser, H., Steinbereithner, K., Wagner, O.: Zur röntgenologischen Kontrolle von Lage und Funktion des Cava-Katheters. Anaesthesist 15, 218 (1966).

380. Porges, P.: Erfahrungen mit der Subclaviapunktion. Klin Med 8, 419 (1966).

381. Porstmann, W.: Fremdkörper im Herz-Kreislaufsystem und ihre transvasale Extraktion mittels Kathetertechnik. Bericht über 15 Fälle. Dtsch Gesundheitsw 30, 1201 (1975).

382. Prout, W.G.: Relative value of central venous pressure monitoring and blood volume measurement in the management of shock. Lancet 1968 I, 1108.

383. Pruitt, B.A., Stein, J.M.: Intravenous therapy in burn patients. Arch Surg 100, 399 (1970).

384. McRae, A.T., Medalle, V.M., Pate, J.W., Richardson, R.L.: Polyethylene catheter embolus. Am Surg 39, 57 (1973).

385. Raffensperger, J.G., Ramenotsky, M.L.: A fatal complication of hyperalimentation. Surgery 68, 393 (1970).

386. Rams, J.J., Daivoff, G.R., V. Mouldner, P.: A simple method for central venous pressure measurements. Arch Surg 92, 886 (1966).

387. Ranninger, K.: An instrument for retrieval of intravascular foreign bodies. Radiology 91, 1043 (1968).

388. Rappaport, A.M., Graham, R.K., Kedrick, W.W.: The use of polyethylene tubing in prolonged intravenous infusions. Can Med Assoc J 72, 698 (1955).

389. Rashkind, J.W.: A cardiac catheter device for removal of plastic catheter emboli from children's heart. J Pediatr 74, 618 (1969).

390. Rea, W.J., Wyrick, W.J., McChelland, R.N., Webb, W.R.: Intravenous hyperosmolar alimentation. Arch Surg 100, 393 (1970).

391. Refetoff, S.: Iatrogenic hydrothorax. Ann Intern Med 63, 327 (1965).

392. Reichelt, A.: Pathomorphologische Beobachtungen nach Anwendung des sogenannten Vena Cava-Katheters. Anaesthesiologie und Wiederbelebung, Vol. 13, Infusionstherapie, Berlin-Heidelberg-New York: Springer 1966.

393. Richardson, J.D., Grover, F.L., Trinkle, J.K.: Intravenous catheter emboli. Experience with twenty cases and collective review. Am J Surg 128, 722 (1974).

394. Richter, G., Ebner, E., Felsch, G., Wesser, M.: Vena-Subclavia-Katheterisierung − infraclaviculär oder supraclaviculär? Dtsch Gesundheitsw 28, 107 (1973).

395. Ricour, C., Nihoul-Fékété, C., Berlin, P.,

Royer, P., Pellerin, D.: Alimentation parentérale continuée par cahtéter intracave chez l'enfant. Ann Chir Infant Parm **13**, 7 (1972).

396. Rolle, J.: Vergleichende Untersuchungen zur Oberflächenbeurteilung von Kunststoffverweilkanülen. Bruns Beitr Klin Chir **219**, 468 (1972).

397. Ronk, R.: Weichmacher im Blut. Eur Med **3**, 22 (1971).

398. Ross, A. M.: Polyethylene emboli: How many more? Chest **57**, 307 (1970).

399. Ross, J. K.: Vena caval infusion. Postgrad Med J **33**, 623 (1957).

400. Ross, S. A.: Infusion phlebitis; selected factors. Nurs Res **21**, 313 (1972).

401. Rossi, P.: "Hook catheter" technique for transfemoral removal of foreign body from the right side of the heart. Am J Roentgenol Radium Ther Nucl. Med **109**, 101 (1970).

402. Royal, H. O., Shieldes, J. B., Donati, R. M.: Misplacement of central venous pressure catheters and unilateral pulmonary edema. Arch Intern Med **135**, 1502 (1975).

403. Ryan, G. M., Howland, W. S.: An evaluation of central venous pressure monitoring. Anaesth Analg Curr Res **45**, 754 (1966).

404. Ryan, J. A.: Catheter complications in total parenteral nutrition. N Engl J Med **290**, 757 (1974).

405. Sabuncu, N., Volles, E., Gressner, P., Prill, A., Harms, U.: Pathologisch-anatomische Befunde und haemodynamische Grundlagen bei Anwendung des Vena subclavia-Katheters. Dtsch Z Nervenheilkd **196**, 266 (1969).

406. Saegesser, M.: Die Bedeutung des zentralen venösen Blutdruckes in der Chirurgie. Schweiz Med Wochenschr **95**, 974 (1965).

407. Salo, E. L., Eerola, R., Eerola, M.: Der Vena-Subclavia-Katheter bei Kindern. Z Kinderchir **12**, 3 (1973).

408. Scebat, L., Renais, J., Meeus-Bith, L., Le Nègre, J.: Accidents, indications et contreindication du cathéterisme des cavités droites du cœur. Arch Mal Coeur **50**, 943 (1957).

409. Schaeffer, H.: Eine neue Methode zur Bestimmung des zentralen Venendruckes beim Menschen. Klin Wochenschr **31**, 802 (1953).

410. Schaeffer, H.: Zur Frage der Vena anonyma-Punktion als Zugangsweg für Infusionen und Transfusionen. Anaesthesist **16**, 303 (1968).

411. Schapira, M., Sterin, W. Z.: Hazards of subclavian vein cannulation for central venous pressure monitoring. JAMA **201**, 111 (1967).

412. Scharf, F. L., Berman, B. J., Cleveland, E. D.: Some complications in the use of indwelling intravenous polyethylene catheters. Med. Serv. J. Can. **15**, 724 (1959).

413. Schechter, E., Parisi, A. F.: Removal of catheter fragments from pulmonary artery using a snare. Br Heart J **34**, 699 (1972).

414. Schlag, G.: Die Bedeutung des zentralen Venendruckes in der Traumatologie. Chirurg **38**, 523 (1967).

415. Schlarb, K.: Subclaviapunktion. Anaesthesist **21**, 477 (1972).

416. Schloßmann, D.: Thrombogenic properties of vascular catheter materials in vivo. Radiology **91**, 251 (1968).

417. Schmidt, Ch., Teucher, H. J.: Die Katheterisierung der Vena subclavia als Bestandteil der Intensivtherapie. Z Aerztl Fortbild **65**, 367 (1971).

418. Schmitz, E. R., Martin, E., Keller, P.: Grundlagen der Venenpunktion. Infusionstherapie **3**, 180 (1976).

419. Schöche, J.: Der Subclavia-Katheter in der chirurgischen Intensivtherapie. Zbl Chir **98**, 270 (1973).

420. Scholz, G., Loewe, K. R.: Die Punktion der Vena subclavia und ihre Komplikationen aus pathologischanatomischer Sicht. Med Welt **20**, 2248 (1969).

421. Schulte, H. D.: Anatomische und technische Möglichkeiten der intravenösen Infusionsbehandlung. Dtsch. Med. Wochenschr. **94**, 1793 (1969).

422. Schumann, G.: Die Komplikationen bei der Anwendung sog. zentraler Venenkatheter aus pathologisch-anatomischer Sicht. Z Kreislaufforsch **60**, 355 (1971).

423. Schweikert, C. H., Gruenagel, H. H.: Doppelseitiger Pleuraerguß bei Infusionstherapie am Hals. Thoraxchirurgie **11**, 421 (1964).

424. Shander, D.: Removal of an embolized polyethylene catheter using an uretral stone catheter. Chest **57**, 348 (1970).

425. Shang, N. G. W., Rosen, M.: Positioning central venous catheters through the basilic vein. A comparison of catheters. Br J Anaesth **45**, 1211 (1973).

426. Shenkin, H. A.: On the diagnosis of hemorrhage in man. Am J Sci **4**, 421 (1944).

427. Siewert, R., Bauers, S., Wiek, K., Bortfeldt, K.: Bakterielle Komplikationen beim Venenkatheterismus. Dtsch Med J **21**, 333 (1970).

428. Silberschmid, M., Saito, S., Smitz, L. L.: Circulatory effects of acute latic acidosis in dogs prior and after hemorrhage. J Surg. **112**, 175 (1966).

429. Simon, J.: Praxis und Technik der parenteralen Ernährung. Prakt Anaesth **11**, 146 (1976).

430. Smith, B. E., Modell, H. J., Gaub, M. L., Moya, F.: Complications of subclavian vein catheterization. Arch Surg **90**, 228 (1965).

431. Smithwick, W., Stalheim, G. K., Love, J. W.: Removal of foreign bodies from the superior vena cava and right atrium without thoracotomy. Ann Thorac Surg **17**, 197 (1974).

432. Smits, H., Freedman, L. R.: Prolonged venous

catheterization as a cause of sepsis. N Engl J Med **276**, 1229 (1967).

433. Smyth, N.P.D., Rogers, J.B.: Transvenous removal of catheter embolism from the heart and great veins by endoscopic forceps. Ann Thorac Surg **11**, 403 (1971).

434. Solassol, Cl., Joyeux, H., Etco, L., Pujol, H., Romien, Cl.: New techniques for long-term intravenous feeding. Ann Surg **179**, 519 (1974).

435. Soni, J., Osatinsky, M., Smith, Th., Vega, S., Vela, J.E.: Nonsurgical removal of polyethylene catheter from the right cardiac cavities. Chest **57**, 398 (1970).

436. Splith, G., Otto, U.: Die Vena subclavia-Punktion. Indikation, Technik und Komplikationen bei 523 Fällen. Z Ges Inn Med **27**, 486 (1972).

437. Stahl, W.M.: Resuscitation in trauma: The value of central venous pressure monitoring. J. Trauma **5**, 200 (1965).

438. Stampfl. B.: Die Endothelialisierung von Gefäßauflagerungen. Verh Dtsch Ges Pathol **46**, 272 (1962).

439. Stein, J.M., Pruitt, B.A.: Cannula sepsis. N Engl J Med **282**, 1452 (1970).

440. Steiner, U.L., Bartley, T.D., Byers, F.M.: Polyethylene catheter in heart; report of a case with successful removal. JAMA **193**, 1054 (1965).

441. Stengert, K., Jurczyk, W., Siennicki, R., Wysocki, E.: Der Zentralvenendruck in der Anaesthesie und der Schockbekämpfung. Anaesthesist **16**, 125 (1967).

442. Stewart, R.D., Stanislow, C.: Silastic intravenous catheters. N Engl. J. Med. **265**, 1283 (1961).

443. Stieber, K.H.: Die unblutige Katheterisierung der Vena cava superior. Med Klin **64**, 388 (1969).

444. Still, V.: Indikation und Durchführung der Katheterisierung der Vena cava cranialis. Wiederbelebung Organers. Intensivmed **7**, 52 (1970).

445. Stöberl, R.: Der sogenannte Cava-Katheter: Technik und eigene Erfahrungen. Wien Klin Wochenschr **68**, 639 (1965).

446. Stoeckel, H.: Kreislaufüberwachung bei Säuglingen und Kleinkindern mit Hilfe des zentralen Venendruckes. Anaesthesist **18**, 250 (1969).

447. Mc Sweeney, W.J., Schwartz, D.C.: Retrieval of a catheter foreign body from the right heart using a guide wire clefelctor system. Radiology **100**, 61 (1971).

448. Sykes, M.K.: Venous pressure as a clinical indication of adequacy of transfusion. Ann Coll Surg Engl **33**, 185 (1963).

449. Tatsumi, T., Howland, W.J.: Retrieval of a ventriculoatrial shunt catheter from the heart by a venous catheterization technique. J Neurosur **32**, 593 (1970).

450. Taylor, F.W.: Catheter embolus. Arch Surg **86**, 177 (1963).

451. Taylor, F.W., Rutherford, C.E.: Accidental loss of plastic tube into venous system. Arch Surg **86**, 177 (1963).

452. Taylor, W.H.: Management of acute renal failure following surgical operation and head injury. Lancet **1957/II**, 703.

453. Teske, H.J., Fassolt, A., Braun, U., Kink, F.: Ergebnisse phlebographischer Kontrolluntersuchungen beim infraclaviculär eingeführten Vena cava-Katheter. Fortschr Geb Roentgenstr Nuclearmed **112**, 189 (1970).

454. Thayssen, P.: Postinfusion phlebitis and the calibre of the catheter. Ugeskr Laeger **135**, 1238 (1973).

455. Thomas, C.S.: Pericardial tamponade from central venous catheters. Arch Surg **98**, 217 (1969).

456. Thomas, D.E., Whittaker, L.D.: Embolization of indwelling venous catheter. Milit Med **135**, 120 (1970).

457. Titone, C., Lefton, Ch., Sakwa, S.: A technique for chronic subclavian vein catheterization. Surg Gyecol Obstet **137**, 489 (1973).

458. Tögel, H.: Seltene Komplikationen nach Anlegung eines Cava-superior-Katheters. Münch Med Wochenschr. **116**, 807 (1974).

459. Tofield, J.J.: A safe technique of percutaneous catheterization of the subclavian vein. Surg Gynecol Obstet **128**, 1069 (1969).

460. Trusler, G.A., Mustard, W.T.: Intravenous polyethylene catheter successfully removed from the heart. Can Med Assoc J **79**, 558 (1958).

461. Tsingoglou, S., Forrest, D.M.: Complications from holter ventriculoatrial shunts. Brit J Surg **58**, 372 (1971).

462. Tsueda, K., Jean-Francois, J.L., Gonzales, E.C.: Connulation of the superior vena cava − a new approach. Anaesthesia **40**, 304 (1974).

463. Tulgan, H., Budnitz, J.: Prolonged survival after catheter embolus. Ann Intern Med **59**, 564 (1963).

464. Turner, D., Sommers, S.C.: Accidental passage of a polyethylene catheter from the cubital vein to the right atrium. N Engl J Med **251**, 744 (1954).

465. Udwadia, T.E., Edwards, A.E.: Accidental loss of plastic tube into the venous system. Br Med J **2**, 1251 (1963).

466. V. Ungern-Sternberg, Fr.W.: Ungewöhnlicher Verbleib eines verlorengegangenen Subclaviakatheters. Chirurg **42**, 331 (1971).

467. Vandeghen, P., Daigneux, D., Musters, A.: Le cathéterisme veineux par la voie sousclaviaire. Rev. Franc. Géront **10** Suppl. 87 (1964).

468. Vaughn, C.C., Rucker, Ch.M., Lee, L.: Trans-

venous removal of broken catheters from the heart and great veins without thoracotomy. Ariz Med **29**, 117 (1972).

469. Verel, D.: Percutaneous intubation of the femoral vein for transfusion. Lancet **1958/I**, 716.

470. Vic-Dupont, J., Cormier, M., Lecompte, Y.: Venous ligature in purulent thrombophlebitis following venous catheter. Chirurgie **99**, 285 (1973).

471. Volles, E., Gressner, P., Dahlmann, W., Prill, A., Subuncu, N.: Der Vena-subclavia-Katheter. Dtsch Med Wochenschr **52**, 2682 (1969).

472. Van Vroonhoven, Th.: Catheterisatie van de vena superior; alternativen voor venasectie. Med T Geneesk **117**, 909 (1973).

473. Vuorinen, J., Helenins, A. S., Kjellberg, M.: Bacteraemia as a complication of subclavian vein catheterization. Ann Chir Gynaecol Penn **62**, 286 (1973).

474. Walter, M. M., Sanders, R. C.: Pneumothorax following supraclavicular subclavian venepuncture. Anaesthesia **47**, 453 (1969).

475. Walters, M. B., Stanger, H. A. D., Rotem, C. E.: Complications with percutaneous central venous catheters. JAMA **220**, 1455 (1972).

476. Watkin, R. R.: The value of central venous pressure measurement during general surgery. Br J Anaesth **37**, 428 (1965).

477. Weber, D., Wittig, D., Uhlmann, B., Reinhard, G., Baumann, G.: Infusions- und Mikrokathetertechnik auf einer internistischen Intensivstation. Ber Ges Inn Med **9**, 248 (1974).

478. Webre, D. R., Arens, J. F.: Use of cephalic and basilic veins for introduction of central venous catheters. Anaesthesia **38**, 389 (1973).

479. Weil, M. H.: Fluid repletion in cerculatory shock. JAMA **192**, 668 (1965).

480. Weissbach, L., Riefl, T.: Ein neues Besteck zur Punktion und Katheterisierung der Vena subclavia. Infusionstheraie **4**, 315 (1973).

481. Weissbach, L., Klippel, K. F.: Der periphere Venenkatheterisierung über eine teilbare Punktionskanüle. Infusionstherapie **1**, 382 (1973/74).

482. Wellmann, K. F.: Polyäthylenkatheter-Embolien. Dtsch Med Wochenschr **92**, 2087 (1967).

483. Wellmann, K. F., Reinhard, A., Salazar, E. P.: Polyethylene catheter embolism. Review of the literature and report of a case with associated fatal tricuspid systemic candidiasis. Circulation **37**, 380 (1968).

484. Wiemers, K.: Postoperative Frühkomplikationen. Stuttgart: Thieme, 1969.

485. Wiggers, C. J.: Physiology of Shock. New York: The Commonwealth Fund, 1950.

486. Wilmore, D. W., Dudrick, St. J.: Prevention of cannular sepsis. Preliminary report. N Engl J Med **277**, 433 (1967).

487. Wilson, J. N., Owens, J. C.: Continous monitoring of venous pressure in optimal blood volume. maintenance. Surg Forum **XII**, 94 (1961).

488. Wilson, J. N.: Central venous pressure in optimal blood volume maintenance. Arch Surg **85**, 563 (1962).

489. Wirbatz, W., Tschirner, L., Meyer, M., Markwart, H. J., Schwarz, H.: Katheterismus der Vena cava mit dem Reservoirkatheter. Dtsch Gesundheitsw **27**, 2101 (1972).

490. Wisheart, J. D., Hassan, M. A., Jackson, J. W.: A complication of percutaneous cannulation of the internal jugular vein. Thorax **27**, 496 (1972).

491. Worms, R.: Les complications septicémiques des cathétérisations intraveineuse prolongées. J. Chir. (Paris) 89, 543 (1965).

492. Wrbltzky, R., Vogel, W.: Zur Technik der infraklavikulären Punktion der Vena subclavia und Indikation des Subclaviakatheters. Z Prakt Anaesthesie **2**, 120 (1967).

493. Yarom, R.: Subclavian venepuncture. Lancet 1964/I 1152.

494. Yoffa, D.: Supraclavicular subclavian venepuncture and catheterization. Lancet 1965/II 614.

495. Zettergoist, E., Carlson, L. A., Liljedahl, S. O.: Influence of indwelling polyethylene catheters on the elimination of 125 g Fibrinogen in bags. Bibl. Anat **10**, 458 (1969).

496. Zimmermann, B.: Scientific apparatus and laboratory methods. Intravenous tubing for parenteral therap. Science **101**, 567 (1945).

Subject Index

Advances in Cardiopulmonary Resuscitation

The Wolf Creek Conference, 1975

Editor: P. Safar
Associate Editor: J.O. Elam

92 figures. XVI, 302 pages. 1977
ISBN 3-540-90234-1

Contents: The Pre-Arrest Period. – Airway Obstruction and Respiratory Arrest. – Circulatory Arrest. – Drugs in Cardiopulmonary Resuscitation. – Electrocardiography, Pacing and Defibrillation. – The Immediate Post-Resuscitative Period. – Special Considerations. – Historic Vignettes.

This book is more than the Proceedings of the Wolf-Creek Conference on Advances in Resuscitation. The 46 papers of this volume have been written by 24 authors, most of whom were first or second generation pioneers of modern resuscitation, which began in the 1950's. The topics include the pre-arrest period, airway obstruction and respiratory arrest; circulatory arrest; drugs in CPR; electrocardiography-pacing-defibrillation, the immediate post-resuscitative period (with special emphasis on recent advances in brain resuscitation); special considerations (such as massive hemorrhage, near-drowning, educational and legal considerations); and historic vignettes. Some of the papers have primarily teaching value; others bring new, as yet unpublished, data, and others are unique because of unpublished historic facts they convey. The historic vignettes and discussions of other papers include stories and quotes of deceased pioneers in resuscitation, such as Claude Beck and William Kouwenhoven. The 24 clinician-scientists who met for this "think tank" pre-distributed manuscripts in order to take account of the present developments in CPR, and to have a look into the future. Their edited manuscripts and discussions published in this volume represent a synthesis of recent scientific, clinical and educational advances of respiratory, circulatory and cerebral resuscitation.

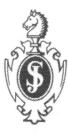

Springer-Verlag
Berlin
Heidelberg
New York

Manual of Critical Care Medicine

Editors: M.H. Weil, P.L. DaLuz

Approx. 68 figures. Approx. 320 pages. 1977
ISBN 3-540-90270-8

Contents: Respiratory Crises. – Shock and Trauma. – Endocrine, Neurological, and Gastrointestinal Crises. – Cardiovascular Crises. – Renal and Metabolic. – Planning and Operations.

This handbook is intended as a resource for physicians, surgeons, and anesthesiologists who serve as clinicians at the bedside of the direly ill and injured. In contrast to more encyclopedic textbooks or literature references that detail the medical, surgical, or anesthesia practice, the focus is on mechanisms, diagnosis, and treatment of immediately life-threatening disturbances. Current guidelines to method of organization and operation of Critical Care Units and methods of patient monitoring are also discussed. In brief, the volume represents an "update" of current practices and therefore is likely to be particulary useful for the clinician who seeks to improve and maintain his competence in critical care medicine. Details of management are given in substantial detail. Together with a carefully prepared index, the volume is therefore anticipated to be of direct value as an immediate reference for patient care in Critical Care Units.

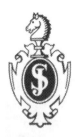

Springer-Verlag
Berlin
Heidelberg
New York